Nu

RT
86
07
1990

Orlando, Ida Jean.

The dynamic nurse-
patient
relationship.

The Dynamic
Nurse-Patient Relationship
Function, Process, and
Principles

Ida Jean Orlando, RN, MA

**Associate Director for Nursing
Education and Research
Department of Nursing
Metropolitan State Hospital
Waltham, Massachusetts**

Pub. No. 15-2341

National League for Nursing

ISBN 0-88737-489-1

This book was set in Garamond by Publications Development Company. The
editor and designer was Allan Graubard. Clarkwood Corporation was the
printer and binder.

The cover was designed by Lillian Welsh.

This book is a reissue of the 1961 edition.

Printed in the United States of America

Contents

Preface to the NLN Edition   **vii**

Preface to the First Edition   **ix**

Acknowledgments to the First Edition   **xiii**

Foreword   **xvii**

1   The Task of the Professional Nurse   **1**

2   The Patient's Distress in Relation to Nursing
Function   **11**

     Physical Limitations   **12**
     Adverse Reactions to the Setting   **17**
     Inability to Communicate Needs   **24**

3   The Nursing Situation in Relation to Principles
of Practice   **31**

     Nursing Data   **31**
     Elements of Nursing Process   **36**

4   Problems in Nursing Situations   **73**

     Development of Nursing Problems   **73**
     Methods of Prevention and Resolution   **90**

Preface to the NLN Edition

If I had been more courageous in 1961, when this book was first written, I would have proposed it as "nursing process theory" instead of as a "theory of effective nursing practice." A "deliberative" process was presented as a guide for nurses to practice "effectively." Conversely, an "automatic" process was shown to be "ineffective." "Effectiveness" was conceptualized and illustrated as "improvement" in the patient's behavior. The "improvement" stemmed from the fact that the deliberative process made it possible for the nurse to identify and meet the patient's *need for help.* (Throughout this text only the phrase *"need for help"* should have been used and not the word *"need."*)

The term *nursing process* has undergone numerous redefinitions, and in some cases the definitions and descriptions pervert the original intent. Definitions by others have no relevance to this work unless the nurse's unique thoughts and feelings that result from perceptions of the patient's behavior are specified.

Published research studies emanating from the Yale School of Nursing in the very early 1960s showed that use of a deliberative process resulted in helpful outcomes. A few years later these studies came to an abrupt halt. However, I continued to develop and refine the formulations contained in this work. The "deliberative process" was renamed nursing process "with discipline," and the "automatic process" was renamed nursing process "without discipline." These changes and other refinements, as well as the objective measures which were developed, were reported in my 1972 publication, *The Discipline and Teaching of Nursing Process: An Evaluative Study*. This work isolated a verbal form of the process discipline which was tested and then evaluated. Only the process discipline was found to have a significant positive relationship to the operational definition of "effective outcome."

Despite the many quantitative positive findings for the verbal form of the process discipline, interest in the work since 1973, in the United States at least, appeared to diminish. Higher price tags were being placed on advanced knowledge in medical fields as well as protocols and educational requirements to follow the new technologies. However, Japanese, Hebrew, French, and Portuguese editions have since appeared with a Dutch edition appearing as late as 1982. I found this encouraging as I am encouraged every day by peers and colleagues I work with at the Metropolitan State Hospital in Waltham, Massachusetts. Nurses are increasingly and in increased numbers taking a firmer stance in assuming authority to find out and meet the patient's immediate needs for help.

Everything in nursing continues to change rapidly as do positions held by professional nurses. What happens between nurses and patients has not changed and that is what this book is all about.

The reissue of *The Dynamic Nurse-Patient Relationship* by the National League for Nursing may well help nurses pick up where the Yale studies left off: resume demonstrating outcomes (often marvelous) as a result of finding out and meeting the patient's immediate needs for help.

Ida Orlando Pelletier
March 1990

Preface to the First Edition

In 1954 the Yale University School of Nursing was awarded a five-year project grant by the National Institute of Mental Health of the United States Public Health Service. The purpose of the project was to identify the factors which enhanced or impeded the integration of mental health principles in the basic nursing curriculum. In carrying out the project, mental health principles in nursing were conceived of as nursing practice which helps patients maintain or restore their sense of adequacy or well-being in stressful situations associated with their illness. Since a person who is ill is likely to have his sense of adequacy or well-being disrupted, it logically followed that all nursing must have a mental health orientation regardless of the patient's illness.

Although this seemed a sound approach, it did not indicate clearly how nursing practices could achieve the desired outcomes. The principles guiding effective practice had first to be identified in order to establish the groundwork for the student's education.

The study was carried out by observing and participating in experiences with patients, students, nurses, service and instructional personnel. At the end of three years, new data brought no further clarification or elaboration of findings which had already been made and it was considered that the study period had ended. Because of this and although the project grant was awarded for a period of five years it was terminated at the end of the fourth year. The last year of the project grant was utilized to formulate the findings of the study, i.e., the content of instruction, the teaching process and the learning environment, needed by students for the development of a professional nursing role. This book contains only the content of instruction. The teaching process and the learning environment will be reported in another book.

The purpose of this book is to offer the professional nursing student a theory of effective nursing practice. It is hoped that the application of this theory will help the student develop her professional role and identity.

The nature of the patient's distress and his need for help are examined in order to identify professional nursing function. The nursing situation is analyzed in terms of its elements (the patient's behavior, the nurse's action and reaction) as they effect the process of helping the patient. From this analysis, principles of effective nursing practice are formulated and then related to: (1) the development of nursing problems (when principles are not applied) and (2) the prevention of nursing problems (when principles are applied).

Recognizing that the nursing profession is currently concerned with nurse-patient relationships, the nurse's professional role and identity, and the development of knowledge which is distinctly nursing, it is believed that this volume can serve as a contribution to these three areas. It identifies the function, process and principles of professional nursing practice; it integrates function, process and principles in practice and may therefore, spell out the distinctive role of the professional nurse; and it may provide a foundation for the systematic study of nursing, i.e., how the nurse effects the patient and the resulting course of the patient's condition.

The theory advocated in this book has been developed from a study of experiences in nursing and teaching. It has been successfully applied in the nursing of patients with medical, surgical, obstetric and psychiatric conditions and is applicable to the nursing of adults and children whether in the home, hospital or clinic. It is hoped that basic students will test it in their own learning experiences and that graduate nurses will test its validity in practice.

Ida Jean Orlando

Associate Professor of Mental Health and Psychiatric Nursing

Director of the Graduate Program in Mental Health and Psychiatric Nursing

Yale University School of Nursing

September 1958

Acknowledgments to the First Edition

I am grateful to all who helped make this work possible, especially the National Institute of Mental Health of the United States Public Health Service. Invaluable assistance was given by the Mental Health Committee of the Yale University School of Nursing which served in an advisory capacity to Marion Russell, Director of the project and Chairman of the Committee until 1957. The Committee included Leo Simmons, Helen Gillmore, Elizabeth Bixler Torrey and Herman Stein. Miss Russell conceived of mental health principles in the basic curriculum as effective nursing education. Her broad vision inspired my task and for her wholehearted support I express my gratitude.

The ideas set forth in this book are not new but the nursing formulations reflect my own synthesis of experience in working and learning with teachers, students, nurses, patients, friends and colleagues. Although their names are too numerous to mention, I am grateful to all who shared with me the experiences which underlie this book. I owe a special debt of gratitude to Florence S. Wald and to Ernestine Wiedenbach for their understanding and encouragement.

My deep appreciation is expressed to Madalon Amenta who helped select the material for the manuscript; to Myrtie

Carpenter for editorial assistance; and to Mary Shaw, Lorraine Johnson and Germaine Boucher for their secretarial help. Special thanks goes to Richard H. Miller, Nursing Editor of G. P. Putnam's Sons, for his unfailing support during the tedious task of preparing the manuscript for press.

I.J.O.

To My Students

Foreword

First published in 1961 and long out of print, *The Dynamic Nurse-Patient Relationship: Function, Process and Principles* remains a book of enduring relevance. Its reissue by the National League for Nursing is thus an occasion of significance. Until now, nurses and nursing faculty interested in Orlando's book have had to rely on secondary sources that provide varying theoretical interpretations only.

Orlando's work was a major force in shifting the nurse's focus from the medical diagnosis to the patient's immediate experience. In her book, Orlando clearly articulates the uniqueness of each patient's immediate need for help as well as the uniqueness of the nurse's deliberative process in determining with the patient his or her specific need. The use of Orlando's theory thus prevents the nurse from acting on invalidated assumptions. Henderson (1978) and other theorists also cite Orlando's theory as emphasizing the necessity of involving patients in all aspects of their care. Nursing care has become more individualized as a result of this involvement.

One special appeal of this book is its simplicity of language. Succinct descriptions of the nursing process express elegantly what nurses perceive as the essence of nursing, namely, determining and meeting, directly or indirectly, the patient's need for help in the immediate nurse-patient contact. The patient's requirement for nursing originates from physical limitations, environmental experiences, and reactions that prevent him or her from clearly communicating distress. Orlando provides numerous situations of how the deliberative nursing process is implemented in practice. Nurses reading this book quickly grasp that the patient is the central focus of Orlando's conception of professional practice. The simplicity of her formulations, however, disguises the complexity of the nurse-patient interaction. The importance of using perceptions, thoughts, or feelings to understand the meaning of the patient's immediate behavior is not something a person does naturally. It must be developed.

Orlando was one of the first to use field methodology to develop her theoretical perspectives long before it was accepted as appropriate. From participant-observer notes, she devised an ingenious conception of the elements and relationships involved as the nurse determines the meaning of the patient's immediate behavior. There is no doubt that Orlando's formulations here have had substantial influence on the nursing education, practice, research, and literature that followed. Barron (1966), Dumas and Leonard (1963), Elms and Leonard (1966), and Tryon (1966) all integrated Orlando's concepts into their groundbreaking studies on patient outcomes.

Although recent research has focused on patient descriptions, there is also renewed interest in what Diers (1987) calls "finding out what in nursing works." This reflects a return to studying what happens to the patient as the result of the nurse's care, the heart of Orlando's work.

The reissue of this time-honored book will inspire a new generation of nurses to use Orlando as the basis for their practice and research. It has served me well and I hope it will do the same for others who are fascinated with the process and outcomes of the nurse-patient relationship.

Norma Jean Schmieding, EdD, RN
Associate Professor of Nursing
University of Rhode Island
Kingston, Rhode Island

REFERENCES

Barron, M.A. (1966). The effects varied nursing approaches have on patients' complaints of pain. *Nursing Research, 15*(1), 90–91.

Diers, D. (1987). Editorial: On research in nursing practice. *Image: Journal of Nursing Scholarship, 19*(3), 106.

Dumas, R.G., & Leonard, R.C. (1963). The effect of nursing on the incidence of postoperative vomiting. *Nursing Research, 12*(1), 12–15.

Elms R.R., & Leonard, R.C. (1966). Effects of nursing approaches during admission. *Nursing Research, 15*(1), 39–48.

Tryon, P.A. (1966). Use of comfort measures as support during labor. *Nursing Research, 15*(2), 109–118.

1

The Task of the Professional Nurse

The preparation of the nurse as a professional person is a difficult task. In a minimum of two and a maximum of five years she must assimilate and apply to practice a wide range of principles from the basic and applied sciences, and all the medical specialties as well as mental health and public health concepts. In one way or another the knowledge she gains is related to people, their environment and their health. Principles and concepts from these other fields enable the nurse to explain her observations of the patient, and the activities which she carries out in relation to them. However, it must be remembered that these principles are derived from the study of particular aspects of the behaving human organism and not from nursing practices as they affect the process of helping the patient. It is important that this distinction be made since general principles which explain behavior or foster health remain valid even when the immediate and individual character of the nursing situation is not considered. However, it is with this specific situation that a nurse must deal.

It is, therefore, exceedingly important for the nurse to distinguish between her understanding of general principles and the meanings which she must discover in the immediate nursing situation in order to help the patient. In making the distinction, the nurse first attempts to understand the meaning to the patient in a time and place context of what she observes and how she can exercise her professional function in relation to it. She also becomes aware of how the patient is affected by what she says or does. This distinction and the importance of having made it can be illustrated.

A Patient Cradles Her Son between Her Knees

"Mrs. Jones, here is your baby. It's your second, isn't it?" Mrs. Jones nodded, pulled herself up in bed, took her son and cradled him between her knees with his head resting on the lower part of her heavy thigh. The nurse handed the bottle to Mrs. Jones, who was telling her son, "There, you can even burp that way." "Oh, no," said the nurse, "We can do that in the nursery, you should hold him close like this. Then when you burp him, hold him over your shoulder. It's important for him to be held and cuddled when you feed him." Mrs. Jones seemed to stiffen as she stared at the nurse and held the baby close. The nurse left.

About five minutes later, Mrs. Jones called out, "Nurse, come quick, my baby is blue!" The nurse ran in, picked up the baby, rushed back to the nursery, gave the baby oxygen and called the doctor. The baby was in good condition, but as a precaution was placed on 24-hour observation in the nursery. The next morning the same crisis arose but with less reaction of alarm. The nurse said, "I'll take the baby to the nursery and have the doctor see him." In the nursery she said to the head nurse, "The baby is all right away from his mother. I think Mrs. Jones rejects her child because she doesn't seem to care if she feeds him or not."

On the third day Mrs. Jones screamed out, "Nurse, come quick, my baby is blue again." This time another nurse tried to find out what was going on before deciding a course of action. The mother held the baby out. The nurse took the baby, noted the fading bluish tinge of his face and hands, and said, "Can you tell me how this happened?" The patient blurted out, "Maybe I held him too tight." "Let's see," said the nurse as she returned the baby to the mother's arms. The patient, leaning over the side of the bed, held the baby with his head crushed against her shoulder and squeezed his armpits as though she were applying tourniquets. The nurse hastened to agree that she did "hold the baby too tight." "But I have to hold him tight or he will fall. Can't I hold him between my legs? That's the way I fed my other baby in bed." "That will protect the baby from falling, and you won't have to hold him tight. Why didn't you feed this baby that way too?" "I thought it was wrong when the other nurse told me to hold him close, and I was afraid to tell her I couldn't." Mrs. Jones positioned the baby, sighed deeply, and said, "Thank you, nurse, I was scared all the other times he turned blue but it didn't scare me this time. Now I can give him the bottle all right."

The understanding required by the nurse, before she could help Mrs. Jones, was distinct from the understanding which would explain her observations and activity. The principles that blueness means oxygen depletion, that babies need tender, loving care, and that the unconscious may be manifest in observed behavior, while valid in themselves, were not sufficient or even appropriate to the unique and immediate experience of the patient and the nurse. What happened between them, how it happened and its relationship to the process of helping the patient was the understanding which was needed.

The principles relative to the depletion and restoration of oxygen and the emotional health of infants were the first which were applied in the situation with Mrs. Jones. The nurses, preoccupied with these applications, were prevented from finding out what was happening to the patient. It was almost as if these principles conditioned the nurses' first thoughts when they observed the patient. Since the principles were valid, the nurses did not find it necessary to question or hesitate in applying them. No nurse would question that babies should be held close, that blue coloring beneath the surface of the skin means oxygen depletion or that Mrs. Jones at some level rejected her child. There are marked and important differences between principles of nursing and principles derived from other fields of theory and practice which have their own distinct aims and responsibilities.

Other fields of theory and practice have developed knowledge which may be used by nurses as needed. In this sense, the broader the nurses' knowledge, the greater are the resources which she may draw upon when necessary in order to help the patient. These are resources for her use in helping people, but they are not principles which guide her practice. A nurse cannot know everything; she may or may not possess the knowledge which is required in a given nursing situation. If she does, so much to her advantage; if she does not, no harm is done as long as she is clear about her responsibility, which is making sure that the patient's requirements are supplied. She may gain the needed knowledge in consultation with other professional people or from the literature.

This point may be further elucidated by examining a situation wherein instruction about the importance of holding babies close was also given.

A Patient Asks a Question

After a nurse instructed a mother on how to hold the baby the mother asked, "Really, nurse, are you sure it's good to hold the baby close?" The nurse was sure, and said so, but also explored the patient's question, "You sound as though you don't believe me?" The patient replied, "I don't know, I want to hold him but mother told me that's the way I spoiled my other baby. He is really spoiled and my mother keeps blaming me for it. She says it's because I held him every time he moved."

The nurse discussed with the patient the difference between holding a baby all the time and at needed intervals. When asked if the explanation made any sense, the patient replied, "Yes, I feel better, because I felt bad about not holding him, he's so little and I would like to. I just won't hold him all the time."

This patient, like Mrs. Jones, needed individual help, not instruction on the importance of holding babies close. She needed help in making a distinction between holding the baby all the time and holding the baby when necessary.

Viewed on a larger scale, both of these illustrations point out the necessity for the systematic study of a nursing situation in order to formulate principles which, when applied to the process of the nurse's activity, can be effective in helping the patient. Learning how to understand what is happening between herself and the patient is the central core of the nurse's practice and comprises the basic framework for the help she gives to patients.

To understand nursing in a professional context, it will be helpful to consider it first in a general sense. It is safe to say that nursing has its roots in the fact that, without help, infants are unable to withstand the environment or take from it what they need. They must have a person who mothers, nurses or cares for them. This concept can readily be translated to the nursing of an adult. An adult at times may find himself in a position not too different from that of a child, and may require the protection or help of one who will care for him. Sometimes his reliance on family or friends is adequate. In this sense, any individual nurses another when he carries, in whole or in part, the burden of responsibility for what the person cannot yet or can no longer do alone.

This rudimentary concept of nursing can be helpful in understanding the meaning of nursing responsibility. It must be kept in mind, however, that nursing as a profession has traditionally aligned itself with the practice of medicine—that art and science which deals with and is responsible for the prevention and treatment of disease. The responsibility of the nurse is necessarily different; it offers whatever help the patient may require for his needs to be met, *i.e., for his physical and mental comfort to be assured as far as possible while he is undergoing some form of medical treatment or supervision.* Some may find this idea unacceptable because the doctor is considered to have the total responsibility for the patient's care. And yet, there is a clear distinction between the medical management of a patient and the way the patient would manage his own affairs and his own comforts if he were able to do so. For instance, when a person says, "I am going to *nurse* my cold," he hastens to arrange his environment so that he can be as free as possible from stress and takes all means at his disposal to increase his comfort. On the other hand, when he says, "I am *doctoring* my cold," we know that he is not only relying on his own inner natural resources, but also on the products of medical science—pills, inhalers and the like.

With these introductory ideas in mind, the framework of the nurse's responsibility must be considered so that the distinctiveness of her task can be understood. It may be assumed that the doctor places the patient under the care of the nurse for either or both of the following reasons: (1) the patient cannot deal with what he needs, or (2) he cannot carry out the prescribed treatment or diagnostic plan alone. As used in this text, *need is situationally defined as a requirement of the patient which, if supplied, relieves or diminishes his immediate distress or improves his immediate sense of adequacy or well-being.*

When the patient is able to meet his own needs and is able to carry out prescribed measures unaided, he is not dependent on the nurse for help. It is not uncommon for patients under medical care to continue their daily living pattern unaided, to take their own medications, to notify the doctor about their complaints, symptoms and the like, to take their specimens to the doctor's office or laboratory, and to study independently ways of fostering their own health. But when the patient cannot meet such needs and when he is not helped, he becomes distressed.

Once agreed that the nurse is responsible for helping the patient avoid or alleviate the distress of unmet needs, it is then important to understand the kinds of experiences which may distress a patient. One might expect that the patient would communicate his distress and need for help in a clear and explicit fashion. Investigation bears out that needs are often unmet because the patient's communication is initially inadequate. Therefore, it is not only important for the nurse to meet the patient's needs but to be able to find out what they are. The patient's distress, his needs, and his inadequate communication, as related to nursing function, will be discussed in Chapter 2.

The distinction which should be made between a principle of nursing and principles of other fields of learning has already been discussed. Whatever principles are brought to bear on the nursing situation, the ultimate aim is to bring about improvement in the nursing care of patients. By definition, *improvement means, to grow better, to turn to profit, to use to advantage.*

Since what a nurse says or does is the exclusive mode through which she serves the patient, then the focus for improvement is what the nurse says or does in practice and how these practices affect the process of care. Understanding how practices help or do not help the patient is the material out of which the nurse develops and improves her knowledge and skill in practice and her professional role and identity.

First consider the practice of observing the patient. A nurse's observations* are the raw material with which she makes and implements her plans for the patient's care. Understandably, the information coming to the attention of the nurse about one patient during the course of a single day can be considerable. Observations which are indirect include hearing comments about the patient at reports or in discussion with doctors, visitors and other service personnel; or through perusal of the doctor's order sheet, progress notes, nurse's notes, etc. Direct observations are acquired from the nurse's own experience with the patient.

The natural consequence of observation is a decision to act or not to act in relation to what is observed. The nurse, herself, may act either with or for the patient, or she may record or report what was observed, what she thought about it and the action she carried out. The records or reports of one nurse are generally brought to the attention of other nurses who may read or hear such things about various patients as, "The intravenous is stopped." "Codeine gr. i for pain." "He's comfortable now." "Instructed on infant care." "He's confused." "He's hallucinating." "Receptive to nurse's suggestions." "Disoriented." "Has not voided." "She slept poorly." "He's complaining of pain." "Catheterized, 600 cc. obtained." "She's divorced." To

---

*Observations comprise all the information pertaining to a patient which the nurse acquires while she is on duty.

the extent that observations such as these are reported or recorded, they comprise nursing data and can be extremely useful to the nurse in her attempts to understand the individual character of the patient's experience.

Basic professional training emphasizes the importance of observation, recording and reporting. They are, therefore, professional practices. In order for these practices to qualify as professional, one must be able to identify how the nurse benefits the patient when she carries them out. To this end, the principle which may guide the nurse in the utilization of nursing data will be discussed in the first section of Chapter 3.

The observation of the patient and the almost infinite variety of activities which nurses carry out need to be studied in relation to one another, that is, as they affect the process of caring for the patient. Otherwise, there appears to be no professional justification for either the observation or the activity.

The focus and stimulus of the professional nurse's service is therefore the patient and his needs. Since the nurse and patient are both people, they interact, and a process goes on between them. The study of what happens, how it happens and its relationship to the process of helping the patient will form the basis for the principles of nursing which will be developed in the second section of Chapter 3.

The discussion of nursing principles which guide effective practice may have some relevance to helping situations in general but they are formulated in ways which relate to the unique context of the nurse's job.

All nursing activities are designed for the benefit of the patient, but sometimes they do not suit the patient because at the same moment he may require something entirely different. When this occurs, the nurse finds that her activity does not achieve the desired result. The distinction between generally useful activities and specific ones which meet the patient's needs, the nature of the conflict and the problems which may come about and a way of dealing with them will be discussed in Chapter 4.

As the examination of nursing data progresses, similar points will be made. But, while similar points may be deduced, they will be derived from the analysis of different nursing practices in order to point out how each practice may be better utilized for the purpose of improving care to patients.

Throughout the text nursing data will be examined, discussed and directed toward the identification of nursing function, process and the formulation of principles of professional nursing practice. A conceptual framework will gradually develop which will suggest the following definition of the purpose and practice of professional nursing.

The *purpose of nursing is to supply the help a patient requires in order for his needs to be met.* The nurse achieves her purpose by initiating a process which ascertains the patient's immediate need and helps to meet the need directly or indirectly. She meets it directly when the patient is unable to meet his own need; indirectly when she helps him obtain the services of a person, agency, or resource by which his need can be met.

The patient's immediate improvement is always relative to *"what was"* when the process started, and is concerned with the patient's increased sense of well-being or a change for the better in his condition. The help received by the patient may also have cumulative value as it affects or contributes toward the individual's adequacy in taking better care of himself.

The nurse, in achieving her purpose, contributes simultaneously to the mental and physical health of her patient. This is so because in helping him she affects for the better his sense of adequacy or well-being. These may be small changes but they are helpful at the moment and may have cumulative value. Nursing in its professional character does not add to the distress of the patient. Instead the nurse assumes the professional responsibility of seeking out and obviating impediments to the patient's mental and physical comfort. In order for the nurse to develop and maintain the professional character of her work she must know and be able to validate how her actions and reactions help or do not help the patient or know and be able to validate that the patient does not require her help at a given time.

Nursing function and the principles which guide it, when integrated in practice, spell out the role of the professional nurse.

2

The Patient's Distress in Relation to Nursing Function

It is helpful to approach the task of identifying professional nursing function on the basis of the current framework of the nurse's responsibility. For specified periods of time the nurse is left with the responsibility of *"watching"* or caring for a patient. It is apparent that all kinds of things happen to patients. Many of their experiences are satisfying; others help them, and still others distress them.

Experiences which are satisfying and helpful to the patient presuppose that his care was at least adequate. However, in assuming the responsibility for optimum care, the nurse must understand how the patient's experiences may interfere with his sense of adequacy or well-being.

It is safe to assume that patients become distressed when, without help, they cannot cope with their needs. Generally speaking, patients require help when their distresses stem from: (1) physical limitations, (2) adverse reactions to the setting, and

11

(3) experiences which prevent the patient from communicating his needs. Each of these will be examined in turn so that a better understanding of the relationship of the patient's distress to his needs and the nurse's function may be established.

PHYSICAL LIMITATIONS

One kind of distress the nurse alleviates or helps the patient avoid is due to his inability to meet needs that he as an individual could ordinarily meet on his own if he were well or in an environment that he was free to control.

In the case of a child, his needs may not be met by himself because he has not yet matured sufficiently; instead he relies on his mother to meet them for him. This point may be illustrated by the reactions of the child who would not eat no matter how the nurse coaxed and loved the child. The child's refusal became more and more insistent. Instead of eating, the child offered the nurses the food. On one occasion a nurse thought the child wanted her to eat. In testing out the thought, she accepted the child's piece of toast and then said, *"Yum, yum."* The child smiled and then ate. It was later learned that the child's mother used this procedure in order to help her child eat.

The patient's complete or partial inability to take care of himself may be due to a temporary or permanent disability, or the setting may restrict him realistically or because he misinterprets it. Each of these circumstances as they pertain to a particular state of distress can be illustrated.

A Patient Makes a Request

For three previous and consecutive mealtimes, a patient did not eat the regular diet which was prescribed for her. At breakfast on the fourth occasion, the nurse thought that the patient was not hungry because she did not begin to eat. The patient said, "Nurse, would you please take away my tray?" The nurse explored the meaning of this request with the patient, and discovered the thought she had about the patient's not being hungry was incorrect. The patient said, "I'm hungry, but I feel sick to my stomach because I didn't have dry toast yesterday morning. I came to the hospital in the middle of the night. I get sick to my stomach and stay that way until I eat dry toast. They gave me buttered toast yesterday, too." "Did you ask for dry toast?" "No," said the patient, "I didn't want to bother the nurses."

When the dry toast was brought and the patient started to eat it, she said, "This does taste good, after no food for 24 hours." Twenty minutes later, the patient ate her breakfast and retained it.

The patient needed dry toast. Before she was hospitalized she was able to meet her own need at home. It is apparent that, if the patient could not move her arms or legs, she would not have been able to get the toast on her own. Nor could she, even if able to, when confined to bed either for diagnostic or treatment purposes, or if patients were not allowed in the kitchen. In any case, someone had to make the toast for the patient. The nurse had to see to it that the patient received the toast and that the hunger and nausea were relieved. On the other hand, suppose that the patient, although willing and able to make her own toast, thought she was not allowed out of bed or in the kitchen. In this case, the nurse would have had to correct the mistaken conclusion before the patient could make her own toast.

Sometimes the nurse finds that she is not free to perform the activity which will meet the patient's need. This is particularly true of the staff nurse who has simultaneous responsibility for many patients. When this is the case, nonprofessional personnel are available and responsible to assist the nurse directly in carrying out her professional concerns and responsibility for the patient's care. The nurse may well have directed a maid to make the patient's toast and perhaps the maid would have even delivered it. Similarly, the patient may require other items which the nurse may prepare and obtain herself or she may inform others about the patient's need. In either case the nurse directly sees to it that the patient's need is met and his distress relieved.

There is, of course, a great deal of variation as to who performs the activity required to help the patient. Whether the nurse does it herself or whether she directs nonprofessional personnel to do it depends on the setting in which she works and the limitations imposed on her activities. For instance, if an individual patient needed help for a walk out-of-doors, a private duty nurse might provide the help herself, whereas a nurse responsible for many patients would have to collaborate with a different person to help the patient take a walk. A distinction should be made between the professional nurse's responsibility *(to ascertain the patient's needs for help and to see to it that they are met)* and the direction of nonprofessional personnel to carry out the activities which meet the patient's needs.

The patient's physical limitations may also prevent him from obtaining the service or help of a different person or agency. The person the patient needs may be one with special skills, training, authority, knowledge, or responsibility, such as a doctor, lawyer, social or welfare worker, minister, etc. or the needed person may be one with whom the patient has a personal relationship, such as a member of the family, friend, etc. Under ordinary circumstances the patient may be perfectly capable of calling in the needed person on his own. However, when the setting, his condition, or his lack of information prevents him from doing so, the nurse may do one of two things, after the need for another person has been identified. She may contact the person or agency or she may inform the patient about the resource but not make the contact herself because the patient is capable of so doing. The course taken by the nurse depends on the patient's capabilities and the nature of his distress. For instance, the nurse may discover that the patient has a new sign or symptom or that an old one has become intensified or may have disappeared. In this instance, the nurse might call the doctor for the patient immediately. On the other hand, the nurse may find that the patient is concerned about the medical advisability of a trip but the patient decides to ask the doctor about it himself when the doctor visits him again.

When the patient needs the help of other people, and for that matter any help, it is important for the nurse to identify the need correctly, because it may at first appear that the patient requires the attention of one person when further exploration reveals that he actually needs the services of someone else. The following illustrates this point.

A Patient "Looks" Sick

Three days had elapsed since the patient gave birth to premature twins. She lay flat on her back and was holding her forehead with her hand. Beads of perspiration covered her face. The nurse asked, "Do you feel sick?" "No," replied the patient, "I'm just a little dizzy. I'm lying flat because sitting makes it worse . . . I'll be all right." Since the nurse didn't think the patient looked well, she said, "You say you'll be all right, but you don't look it to me now . . ." The patient stared at the nurse and paused for a second before saying, "Nurse, my babies are in that room." The nurse did not know what the patient had in mind and asked, "Which room?" "In the room where they charge 16 dollars a day each," replied the patient. Suddenly her face flushed; she sighed and swallowed hard. It seemed to the nurse that the patient wanted to cry, and, to see if that was correct, she asked, "Is that why you look like you want to cry?" The patient nodded, and as tears welled in her eyes, she said, "How am I ever going to pay for it? If the babies are going to be in there for two months, I can't even add up how much it's going to cost." The nurse asked if the patient had talked to anyone about it. "There was no one I could tell. All I could see was the miserable look on my husband's face. He's sicker with worry than I am."

The nurse thought that someone in the business office could help, since neither of them knew what the exact daily charges were or what the patient's hospitalization insurance covered. When the nurse asked the patient if calling the business office seemed like a reasonable next step, the patient said, "Yes, at least I will know where I stand."

The person in the business office informed the nurse that the problem had already been anticipated and funds were available for which the patient's husband was eligible. These funds covered the entire cost of the hospitalization for the premature infants from the date of the mother's discharge. The office had just called in the patient's husband to make application.

The nurse returned and informed the patient about the arrangements. Abruptly the patient sat up, sighed, then said, "Oh, what a relief. I was nearly crazy trying to multiply 32 times 60." In order to be sure the patient was feeling better, the nurse asked, "How is the dizziness?" "It's all gone—I feel better and want to get out of bed now. As a matter of fact, I think I feel strong enough to go home right this minute."

If the nurse had called the doctor before she understood the reason for the dizziness, and the doctor prescribed on the basis of the symptom alone, the patient would not have been relieved of her distress. On the other hand, if the nurse had not been successful in ascertaining the meaning of the complaint or if the patient could attach no meaning to it, the doctor would have been notified in order to safeguard the patient's medical condition.

Before the nurse discovers which person the patient needs he undergoes what can be loosely termed a *"double dose"* of distress; the distress itself and his inability to take steps to relieve it. The next case example will point this out.

A Patient Complains of Pain

A patient complained, "Nurse, I have pain around my stitches." As the nurse draped the patient's abdomen, she asked, "Can you tell me what the pain is like?" The patient sighed deeply and replied, "It's terrible; it isn't exactly sharp—it's more like a throb, but it kept me awake all night. I had stitches before and I felt them, but they felt different." As she examined the stitch area, the nurse said, "It is red and looks harder than it should. I think the doctor should see it. Do you have any objection to my calling him?" "Oh, yes, please call him. He'll do something, I'm sure, and maybe I can get some sleep."

The doctor was notified, and when he examined the area he told the patient, "You have a little infection; nothing to worry about. We'll give you medicine for it and for your pain." "I'm not worried, doctor, I just want the throb to go away so I can sleep. Thanks a lot."

The doctor left, and, as the nurse helped the patient resume his sitting position, the patient said, "You are wonderful. I feel better already." Because the nurse was perplexed, she said, "I don't understand . . . I haven't done anything for your pain yet . . ." "Now, don't misunderstand me, nurse. I still have the pain, although somehow it isn't as bad. You see, I told several nurses my stitches hurt and they told me in one way or another, even though they were very good about it, that pain was to be expected. I was beginning to think I was crazy. I was sure something was wrong. What I mean is . . . it's a relief to know I really was right after all."

This anecdote introduces a second way in which the patient may become distressed: by reacting adversely to an experience in the medical setting. Presumably, some nurses told the patient his stitch pain was to be expected. This was misinterpreted by the patient to mean that what he thought was *"wrong"* was expected by them. Yet the nurses didn't know he thought something was wrong. The patient thought something was wrong on the basis of his previous experience with stitches. When he was told that pain was to be expected, he not only felt he might be crazy, but it somehow also made his pain worse. It is reasonable to assume that the patient would not have felt he might be crazy if he knew exactly what the expected pain was or if he had the courage to question what he was told. Had he understood or felt courageous enough to do this without help, he would have clarified matters by himself.

ADVERSE REACTIONS TO THE SETTING

The patient's reactions in the setting which may cause him distress are generally based on an inadequate or incorrect understanding of an experience in the setting. The distress may come about because the premise upon which the reaction is based is essentially incorrect. The misunderstanding may pertain to the illness, or to preventive, diagnostic or treatment measures, or to something in the environment, or to the activity, authority or responsibility of service personnel and other people.

The important point for consideration is that a patient may react with distress to any aspect of an environment which was designed for therapeutic and helpful purposes.

The following case examples will show how adverse reactions precipitate a patient's need for help and if the help is not forthcoming, the reaction may harm the patient. First an illustration as to how a patient may become distressed through some misunderstanding about his illness.

A Patient Asks for a Bedpan

The patient put her call light on every half hour saying each time, "Can I have the bedpan, nurse?" Nurses responded each time. Sometimes the patient voided and sometimes she did not. On this particular occasion, the nurse said, "I notice you ask for the bedpan more often than most patients, and it's difficult for me to understand because sometimes you pass your water and sometimes you don't. Do you have any idea why?" "Maybe it's because I'm nervous, nurse." "Can you tell me why?" "Whenever I'm nervous, I always feel like I have to pass my water. I wasn't afraid before, but now I think I might have a bad disease. The doctors haven't told me anything yet. Maybe they don't want to upset me. If it wasn't a bad disease they would have told me." The nurse knew that the diagnostic procedures had not yet been completed and that the lab reports were yet to be returned, and explained this to the patient. The nurse asked if the patient still felt nervous. "No, nurse, not now. I figured it must be a bad disease because they did a lot of tests and haven't told me anything. I can wait until they know."

The patient stopped asking for the bedpan at half-hour intervals.

The patient, in waiting for some information about the results of tests, assumed that she had not been told about them because she had a fatal disease. The patient needed to have her mistaken conclusion corrected. When this was done, the patient's discomfort subsided and she stopped asking for the bedpan.

Another patient became distressed because of a false reaction to his environment.

A Patient "Looks" as though He Wants Something

A patient walked to and fro across his room and always in front of the empty chair at the bedside. He would stop instantaneously when he reached the chair, mumble something and then continue walking. The nurse said, "I notice when you reach the chair you stop and it looks as though you want something. Do you?" "Yeah, I want to sit down. I'm dead tired." "Then why don't you?" "Because somebody is in it." "I don't understand. I don't see anyone there, but are you saying that you do?" "Don't get me wrong. I don't see anyone there, I just feel someone is. It's as if you sat in that chair, right now, and then got up. I couldn't sit in it because I would feel you were still there and it would be like sitting in your lap."

Suddenly, the patient grinned. The nurse asked if he could tell her why he was grinning. "It's funny, that's why. Just talking about it doesn't make it half as bad. See, I can even sit now." "I'm so glad," said the nurse, "perhaps we can talk about it each time it happens." "Yeah, I could talk to you all right, but I just can't tell it to anybody. I know it's crazy, but with some people you just don't tell them because they make you feel even crazier. That's the way the world is—some people understand and some don't."

Several weeks later the patient said at one point in a discussion with the nurse, "I'll be okay; I've got three nurses now that I can talk with when it happens. If they aren't here when it happens, instead of walking around the chair killing time all day, I'll say to hell with it and go down and play a game of pool."

The patient was unable to sit in the chair because of his false reaction to it. Not seeing someone in the chair, but feeling that someone was, precipitated his need to talk and feel accepted in spite of his hallucination *(tactile)*. When the need was met, the patient felt better.

A nurse may find that a patient becomes distressed during or after an experience with her or any other person in the setting. As mentioned earlier, any adverse reaction stems from the patient's inadequate or incorrect understanding of his experience. Those in reaction to people in the setting may pertain to their activities, authority or responsibility. Misunderstanding the authority or responsibility of service personnel is more closely related to the development and maintenance of a professional relationship and will be discussed later.

It is reasonable to assume that any activity performed with or for the patient is designed, at least ultimately, for the patient's benefit. But, it sometimes happens that professional and non-professional personnel alike carry out activities which not only do not help the patient but may even hinder his progress. The point of the matter is not whose activity precipitates the patient distress, but that when the patient reacts adversely he needs the help of a nurse—the one who is there caring for him.

A Patient Asks a Question

The patient smiled as two nurses entered her room. One nurse said, "We're going to get you out of bed now," as she proceeded to drape a chair and move some furniture about. The patient smiled, hesitated, bit her lip, then said, "What am I going to do without nurses around?" "You'll manage fine when you go home." Suddenly the patient's face flushed; her respirations quickened. She sighed deeply and closed her eyes as she let her head fall forward. The second nurse thought, then asked, "Do you feel weak?" "No . . . I'm dizzy and I have a headache." The first nurse replied, "Getting out of bed will help you feel stronger," as she proceeded to instruct the patient about getting out of bed. The patient's respirations quickened even more; her lips quivered as she said, "Will I . . . have to go . . . to the clinic . . . when I go home?" The first nurse replied, "Before you leave the hospital you'll get an appointment slip." "Am I all well now, nurse?" As both nurses helped her to the chair, the patient held her hand over her eyes. *(It may be observed that the patient's verbal and nonverbal behavior indicated increased stress, that her questioning behavior was repetitive and it did not change.)*

The second nurse asked, "Why do you want to know if you're well now?" The patient sighed deeply and answered, "Because I don't feel strong enough to go home yet." The first nurse replied, "You're not going home now; it will take several weeks to regulate your insulin and diet." Suddenly the patient smiled; her head became erect and her breathing slower, even though she had exerted herself getting to the chair. Thinking that the patient was feeling better and wanting to check this impression, the second nurse asked, "It looks like what the nurse just said helped you. Did it?" The patient smiled and said, "Yes, nurse, I thought they were sending me home and it's too soon—I've only been here two days and I'm not strong enough yet. They get you out of bed just before they send you home, and the doctors promised they would make me feel strong first. I was afraid because there's no one at home to care for me, and I can't manage by myself yet." Before the nurse left she asked, "How's the dizziness and headache?" "It's all gone. I'm all right now. I was just worried because I couldn't manage by myself yet."

When the nurse told the patient "We're going to get you out of bed," the patient reacted automatically and attached her own meaning to the experience. This reaction distressed the patient and precipitated her need to understand that getting out of bed did not mean she was ready for discharge. When the need was met, the condition of the patient improved.

Nurses are not the only ones who affect patients but they are the ones who carry the continuous responsibility for a patient's care. Therefore, it is the nurse's responsibility to help the patient even if it is not her activity which adversely affects the patient. This does not mean that she is responsible for the activities of other professional persons. An additional example involving the separate activities of a doctor and a nurse might make this clearer. The doctor informed the patient about the kind of anesthesia she would receive; the nurse informed the patient about the time she would be going to the operating room.

A Patient "Looks" as though She Wants Something

It was 9 A.M. From the doorway the nurse saw the patient suddenly lift her head from the pillow. The nurse entered and said, "Do you want something?" The patient's face flushed and her mouth quivered in spite of the obvious attempt to hold her lips together. A few seconds passed before the patient replied, "I don't know. Are they going to send me to the operating room this morning? I had a spell *(epileptic seizure)* last night and they may have changed their minds." "Do you want to know if you are going?" "Please, nurse, find out if I'm going." "Well, I do know that you will be going to the operating room at 10:30 A.M." The patient smiled nervously, and as she thanked the nurse her mouth and hands quivered even more. "It looks as if I've upset you more by telling you the time. Am I wrong?" The patient nodded as tears welled up in her eyes. The nurse asked the patient if she could tell her why she was crying. "I thought maybe they wouldn't send me to the operating room—it's the spinal I'm afraid of, nurse. I was awake all night worrying about it—the doctor said it's the only anesthesia I can have." The patient swallowed hard, then said, "God will help me to be brave." In order to understand why the patient was afraid the nurse asked, "Do you know why you are afraid of a spinal?" "My brother-in-law has had three spinals and he has pain night and day. He has kept my sister awake at night with it for two years now." The nurse couldn't understand the connection, so she continued to explore. "I don't understand—why did your brother-in-law have spinals?" "He had three operations when he broke his back." The nurse asked, "Wouldn't the pain be from the broken back?"

Suddenly the patient's expression changed as she exclaimed, "Oh, God, thank you, nurse. I see God sent you to me now." The nurse tried to clarify the point, but the patient kept interjecting, "Oh, thank God, thank you, nurse. Hand me my rosary beads so I can thank God for sending you to me now. I know I won't get the *"spell"* now." "How do you know that?" "Because I only get them when I'm very nervous—like I was now . . . I can feel them coming; that's why I'm so thankful. If I didn't get the *"spell"* now, I won't have it in the operating room." "If you should get nervous again, do you think you will be able to ask for help?—You will be awake you know?" "Oh, yes, nurse. I can do it because the doctors were very nice to me last night. They explained it all—but I was so afraid when I heard the word *'spinal'* that I couldn't listen."

The patient's face was no longer red, her mouth was no longer quivering, and her facial expression was full of relief as she said, "I'm going to be all right now. I'm not afraid of the operation. I've had operations before and I've been waiting for this one a long time so my urine won't leak. One of my sons is very good to me. He wants to take me out for rides on Sundays, but I can't go because I'm ashamed when my urine leaks. After the operation I can enjoy my Sundays with him." It was 9:15 when the nurse left.

When the doctor informed the patient that she would have a spinal, the patient automatically reacted with fear. The reaction precipitated her need for help in correcting the thoughts which caused the fear. When the need was met, the patient's condition improved.

It might be well to consider briefly what is commonly referred to as *"psychological preparation of the patient"* for operative and treatment procedures and their resulting *"reactions."* The attitude of the patient toward the operation in this illustration was positive and not negative as one might be inclined to think. Her reaction was specifically to the word *"spinal,"* and therefore helping her before the operation had to be specifically geared to her need. It is apparent that an explanation of the operative procedure would not have helped the patient. Again it is necessary to identify the patient's need correctly.

The nurse's professional concern for the patient centers on experiences which may distress him when he cannot cope with his physical limitations, when things go wrong with his medical condition or social situation, or when he misunderstands some aspect of the setting in which he is being treated and cared for. These distresses seem unrelated, and, strictly speaking, they are. However, they have one common feature—they may occur during the time the nurse is responsible for the patient's care. In the light of the foregoing discussion the professional function of the nurse may be stated. *It is the nurse's direct responsibility to see to it that the patient's needs for help are met either by her own activity or by calling in the help of others.* Needs that the patient can meet comfortably on his own would not be of any professional concern to the nurse.

It is important for the nurse to concern herself with the patient's distress because the treatment and prevention of disease proceeds best when conditions extraneous to the disease itself and its management do not cause the patient additional suffering. The disease and its treatment deplete the patient's inner resources and are sufficient for him to cope with. In a way, the nurse focuses her attention on anything that may interfere with his mental and physical comfort. The success of treatment or preventive measures ultimately rests on the patient's own capacity to use them. This is the reason for nursing's traditional and current focus on the importance of helping patients with their needs. How the nurse affects the patient and how this influences the course of the patient's condition have not been systematically studied to any great extent. This area is one of the most promising in the further development of nursing research.

INABILITY TO COMMUNICATE NEEDS

What does the nurse need to know in order to carry out her function of meeting the patient's needs? She must first realize that the patient cannot clearly state the nature and meaning of his distress or his need without her help or without her first having established a helpful relationship with him. The nurse observes the patient's presenting behavior, the meaning of which she cannot understand without further exploration. Some of the examples cited thus far may serve to illustrate this point. *"Nurse, come quick—my baby is blue"* did not automatically mean, *"Maybe I hold the baby too tight."* *"Nurse, would you remove my breakfast tray?"* was very different from *"I'm sick to my stomach because I need dry toast."* *"I'm a little dizzy, nurse"* did not automatically mean, *"I'm worried sick over finances."* The patient who requested a bedpan every half hour did not spontaneously say, *"I'm afraid I have a bad disease."* The patient who walked to and fro in front of his chair did not automatically let anybody know that he needed someone who would talk to and be interested in him in spite of his hallucination.

To the inexperienced person it seems unreasonable for the patient not to ask for the help he needs, since this is the very reason why nurses are available. To those acquainted with psychodynamic concepts it should come as no surprise that people are ambivalent in relation to their dependency needs. It has already been stressed that, from a nursing point of view, it is the meaning to the patient which must be ascertained so that the nurse can be of help.

When the nurse asks the patient why he did not express his distress or need clearly at the onset, she finds that he has his own reasons. Generally speaking, these reasons show that the patient does or says what he thinks is *"right"* or expected of him instead of what he wants for himself.

When the nurse begins to search for the patient's reasons, it is not unlikely that she will think the patient is being unreasonable. However, sufficient exploration will make it possible for her to reverse her judgment.

A Patient "Looks" as if He's in Pain

The patient's position in bed was rigid. He was squinting; a barely perceptible grunt was heard from his tightly closed lips. The nurse asked, "Are you in pain?" The patient sighed deeply, swallowed, and cried. Through his sobbing he said, "I've been in pain for three days now." "Have you told anyone about it?" "No .. . . I didn't tell them because they knew but didn't give me anything." "How did they know if you didn't tell them?" "They knew because the doctor told them right in front of me— that I should have an injection when I told him I was in pain. The head nurse was standing right there when he told them on rounds that I could have it every four hours, but nobody brought it to me. Besides, it isn't right that I should tell on the nurses. Anyway, I didn't want to complain because it isn't my place to tell them what to do."

The initial inability of the patient to communicate clearly his distress or need must be examined further, not only because the restoration of his comfort is delayed but because the inadequate communication of the distress may also seriously threaten his condition. For example:

A Patient Suddenly Jumps

A nurse was asked to help support a patient on her side as another nurse made the bed. Without thinking the nurse placed her hand on the patient's buttock. The patient jumped suddenly.

"Why did you jump like that?" "Because it's killing me and it's getting worse all the time." "*It*" was pain in the perineal region. The nurse saw the left labia and perineum extensively swollen and visibly growing in size. The nurse said, "It looks awful—I think the doctor should see it. Is that all right with you?" "Oh, yes, nurse, please—he'll do something—it's terrible."

While one nurse summoned the doctor to see the hematoma, the other asked, "How were you able to stand the pain when we started to make the bed?" "I don't know, nurse—I couldn't sleep all night. Thanks for helping me." "For what? You still have the pain," said the nurse. "Well, I don't feel like a lunatic now. I told the night nurse this morning that my stitches hurt, but she said they would hurt a little." "Did you tell the night nurse that it wasn't just a little?" "Oh, no, I didn't want to be a baby."

What was happening to both patients or what the patients really meant was not automatically communicated to the nurse. How was the nurse to know the patient was in pain if he deliberately delayed for three days in telling her? How was the nurse to know the patient's stitches hurt a *"lot"* unless the patient specified the intensity of the pain. After all, stitches do hurt a *"little."*

The one patient didn't tell the nurse her stitches hurt more than a *"little"* because she didn't want to be a baby. The other patient didn't tell the nurses about his pain because he felt it wasn't right. The reasoning of both patients was incorrect. The nurse had to correct in some way the patient's mistaken conclusions before she could begin to be of help. It is important to emphasize that while reasons such as these are rationalizations they do in fact prevent patients from disclosing their actual distress or need. Generally, the reason why the patient does not tell the nurse may be traced to the initial nurse-patient relationship. When the nurse and patient first meet they are strangers to each other. Without an actual experience of having been helped the patient doesn't know in any real way that the nurse will help him. He only guesses as to how reliable she is. Without her helpful demonstration, the patient does not clearly understand the nurse's professional function, authority or responsibility in relation to his needs for help. Although she is a stranger, she is professionally prepared and responsible to help him communicate his needs and to see to it that they are met. It is this help which provides the guidelines of their interaction and forms the basis of the nurse-patient relationship.

The initial inability of the patient to communicate the specific meaning of his behavior or what he needs points to two aspects of the nurse's function. First, *the nurse must take the initiative in helping the patient express the specific meaning of his behavior in order to ascertain his distress.* Second, *she must help the patient explore the distress in order to ascertain the help he requires for his need to be met.*

When the nurse begins to explore the meaning to the patient of what has been observed, the patient will more often than not experience the willingness and concern of the nurse because she is in the very process of finding out how she can be of help. In the event that the patient misunderstands the nurse's inquiry, the nurse would have to correct the patient's mistaken idea. Once the patient has been helped, he feels safer to communicate the distress of which he is aware. Interestingly enough, once he trusts the nurse, his communications are more explicit and he is more likely to spontaneously discuss the experiences which distress him. The situation which follows will show how this may occur. It illustrates the patient's extreme reluctance to express his distress or need and how his reluctance may persist until he recognizes through something the nurse does that she is willing to help him. This patient was particularly interesting because the nurse was almost convinced that he was the first she had ever met who stated his need clearly at the onset without assistance or a previous experience of having been helped by her.

A Patient Asks a Question

The patient was a retired university professor who had taught in an American school abroad and who had never previously been ill. According to the nurses, he was "appreciative, distinguished, cooperative, and very polite—He even thanks you when you say good morning."

As the nurse was serving breakfast, the patient asked, "Can you tell me what the ratio is of nurses to patients?" The nurse was about to explore why the patient asked the question, but was interrupted by his giving her a letter from his daughter-in-law who directed a nursing school in a foreign country. "My daughter-in-law wants to know about the hospital's organization, administration and teaching programs." The nurse believed that the patient needed information to answer his letter. She had no reason to think otherwise, since he appeared comfortable as he ate. When the nurse replied, "I don't know what the ratio is, but perhaps . . ." the patient interjected, "I can ask the supervisor tomorrow—she visits me every day. Would you then be so gracious as to tell me which nursing schools affiliate here?"

As the nurse named the schools, the patient suddenly stopped eating, turned his head and stared out the window. The nurse thought the patient was not listening. However, she did not follow up this thought, but instead said, "Didn't you ask for this?" *(This question was almost pointless since the nurse and patient knew he did.)* "Yes, please do go on."

The nurse tried to find out why the patient looked distracted without ascertaining if he actually was. She thought his reaction had something to do with his breakfast tray, but her question did not indicate her thought. "Do you have everything you want?" Without hesitation the patient replied, "Yes, thank you very much for your interest." Without clearly stating her doubts, the nurse persisted, "Are you sure you have all you want?" With some hesitancy the patient replied, "Yes, thank you just the same." Thinking that the hesitancy indicated the patient did want something, but not questioning him directly about it, the nurse replied, "I can get more milk, toast or anything else you would like." The patient sighed, hesitated, then said, "It would be very nice if you could get me more milk, that is, if it isn't too much trouble."

The nurse left to get the milk but became involved in a discussion. However, she did return with the cold milk. Eager to return to the discussion, she hurriedly acknowledged the patient's many thanks. Almost immediately after she left the patient's room she saw his call light go on. She quickly returned and saw that the patient had altered his position in bed and thrown his bed clothing off. His breakfast tray was pushed aside, he was panting and his face was red. He burst out, "Will you please help me?" In a trembling voice he added, "I can usually control myself, but I cannot tolerate this another moment. I did so want to ask you while you were here, but I just couldn't. I do wish you would help me now." As the nurse draped the patient he continued, "They took my tube out yesterday morning, and I've been dribbling ever since. I was extremely uncomfortable all night." He handed the nurse his pajama bottom. It and the drawsheet were drenched with serosanguineous urine. "How is it that someone didn't help you sooner?" asked the nurse as she washed the patient. "I just didn't want to bother the nurses—they are kind and have so much to do." As the nurse rinsed the bath basin, the patient spontaneously said, "These past few minutes are the most enjoyable I've spent in the hospital; cold milk was the only good thing on my breakfast tray. For some reason or other you know what I need almost before I ask, but I'll ask anyway. Would you put the bed down, please? Since you made me feel so well, I would like to sleep now because I didn't all night." The patient slept for several hours.

The nurse was available and willing to help but the patient did not know this in any real way at the onset of their interaction. Eventually, although fortuitously, the patient did get the nurse's message after she insisted on getting him more milk. Her persistence in "doing something" for him made him know that she was available to help him. Only then was he able to spontaneously express his distress. After the nurse met his need he told her, without any hesitation this time, about the last bit of help he needed in order to fall asleep.

Thus, before the nurse establishes her relationship to the patient he does not clearly tell her about his distress or needs; he cannot do so without her help and he does not do so until he is sure she will meet them. Once the relationship is established, his communications to the nurse become clearer and more explicit. When he spontaneously informs the nurse about the specific nature of his distress or what he needs, the nurse can be fairly certain that her professional relationship is established. However, this is not enough. The nurse has other concerns to deal with in maintaining the relationship but these will be discussed later.

More can be said about the illustration just cited. It is understandable that the nurse allowed herself to be convinced that the patient needed answers to his questions, because he was an academic person, he did have a letter from a director of nurses, and without appearing to be distressed was asking questions in order to answer his letter. Despite this amount of evidence, the nurse did not feel completely satisfied when she answered his questions because he seemed inattentive. She sensed that something was wrong but didn't know exactly what it was. Instead of asking the patient about her presumptions, she acted them out. She thought the patient wanted something but did not first check on what it was. Instead, she assumed it might be more food. This kind of nondescript awareness is often referred to as a nurse's intuition. This situation may well illustrate that a nurse's intuition is not a magical quality but rather the thoughts which occur to her in response to direct observations. For example, the nurse in this situation sensed that things were not completely right at the moment she started to answer the questions because the patient's behavior changed dramatically, *i.e., he stopped eating, he looked out the window, and he hesitated in answering her.* This behavior was in marked contrast to his previous attentiveness and matter of fact manner.

The patient's distress as it relates to his needs for help has been examined in order to identify the function. In summary, nursing function and two of its aspects can be restated. *It is the nurse's direct responsibility to see to it that the patient's needs for help are met, either directly by her own activity or indirectly by calling in the help of others.* In order to meet the patient's needs, the nurse *(1) initiates a process of helping the patient express the specific meaning of his behavior in order to ascertain his distress and (2) helps the patient explore the distress in order to ascertain the help he requires so that his distress may be relieved.*

3

The Nursing Situation in Relation to Principles of Practice

NURSING DATA

There are essentially four practices which are basic to nursing: (1) observation, (2) reporting, (3) recording, and (4) actions carried out with or for the patient. These practices should be examined in terms of the benefits gained by the patient when they are carried out.

In the current organization of nursing services it is not possible, or even necessary, for the nurse to spend every moment with the patient except in special instances. However, observations of one kind or another are always available. Observations have been defined as any information pertaining to a patient which the nurse acquires while she is on duty. From this point of view the observations, actions, and reports, or records of other nurses which come to the individual nurse's attention would also be included. These available nursing data may be thought of as the raw material out of which the nurse plans and carries out her concerns for the patient's care.

The observations of an individual nurse may, therefore, be direct or indirect. *Indirect knowledge of the patient consists of any information which is derived from a source other than the patient. This information pertains to, but is not directly derived from, the patient.* Ordinarily, it consists of comments offered by people *(nursing service personnel, other service personnel, other professional personnel, friends and relatives of the patient, etc.)* purposefully and incidentally, formally and informally, at reports, conferences and the like. These comments might consist of observations, judgments, incidents, symptoms and complaints pertinent to the patient. Other indirect sources might include nurses' notes, progress notes, doctors' orders, etc.

Direct knowledge may be described as any perception, thought, or feeling the nurse has from her own experience of the patient's behavior at any or several moments in time. And, of course, the nurse is always in a position to know directly what she said or did with or for the patient.

The nurse devotes a considerable amount of time to acquiring both direct and indirect information about patients, and therefore has at her fingertips an enormous amount of such material. In this respect she has an advantage over other professional people who are *"not around,"* so to speak, to learn as much about the patient. The hospital nurse is in a rather unique position in the professions, because her responsibility for the patient is direct and continuous, extending, on the average, over a period of eight hours per day. Collectively, hospital nurses are responsible for patients over the 24-hour period. This unique position emphasizes the importance of this question: How may the patient derive maximum benefit from the nurse's almost constant practice of observation? The discussion in this section is mostly related to information the nurse acquires indirectly, since what happens in her direct experience with the patient is given emphasis throughout the text.

The direct and indirect observations of the nurse apart from purposeful investigation in an immediate nurse-patient situation are not adequate for the individual nurse to carry out her responsibility of helping the patient with his needs. With this idea in mind and the use of two illustrations, it is possible to discuss the relation between anything a nurse knows about a patient and its usefulness in discerning his needs.

The following situation, in which nurses obtained information indirectly at morning report, illustrates that unless the nurse persists in finding out more about what she learns from someone else, the patient derives no benefit from her having acquired the information in the first place.

A Nurse Hears a Report on Mrs. Smith

A night nurse said at the 7 A.M. report, "Mrs. Smith thought she was going to the bathroom too often. I don't know why because she voided quantity sufficient for me." The day nurse did not use this information in the process of giving the patient morning care. However, at 11:40 A.M. Mrs. Smith complained of *"pain"* to the nurse who had cared for her. Exploration of how the patient experienced the pain brought forth, "It isn't really pain, it's like a pressure feeling down below. I spent most of the night going to the toilet. I felt like I had to have a bowel movement, but I was afraid to push too hard for fear of hurting my stitches." As the situation worked out, the pressure was due to vaginal sponges, which when expelled relieved the patient's *"pain."*

While the information offered at 7 A.M. did not prove to be immediately useful, we cannot discount its potential value at that time. The patient's statement that she was *"going to the bathroom too often"* did not enable the nurse to understand that the patient felt *"pressure"* and needed relief. The information could have been useful in helping the patient sooner had the day nurse found out more about what she heard from the night nurse. Let us assume for a moment that Mrs. Smith did not complain of *"pain"* to the day nurse. The day nurse then would have only known that the patient felt she was *"going to the bathroom too often."* It would seem reasonable to infer that, if the day nurse said to the patient, "The night nurse told me you thought you were going to the bathroom too often, can you tell me why?", then the feeling of *"pressure"* might have become known and the patient would not have complained of *"pain"* later.

The following more detailed illustration shows how indirect knowledge used with the patient may immediately lead to an understanding of the patient's need.

A Nurse Hears Some Comments about a Patient

Over a period of two days several nurses and a doctor were heard making the following comments about a patient. "She refuses to accept any suggestions from the nurse, and I'm concerned that her nipples will break down." "She won't listen when I tell her that her milk isn't in yet." "I don't think she likes the American way of doing things." "I told her yesterday that if she doesn't stop putting the baby to her breast every five minutes her nipples will break down." "She puts the baby to her breast every five minutes and it's like talking to a wall to tell her to stop." "Maybe she doesn't understand because she's only been in the States a year." Another nurse responded to the last comment by saying, "She understands English very well. She just doesn't want to listen."

On the third day a nurse went to see the patient to try to find out what actually was going on. The nurse started out by saying, "Some of the nurses mentioned that you are putting the baby to breast every five minutes. They think you hear what they tell you, but ignore what they say. Is this so?" In broken English the patient replied, "The doctor . . . the nurse . . . they tell me that it hurt my nipples, but I no care—I'm afraid my baby starve—he's hungry! I know I no got enough food—my milk not in yet—baby is hungry, but this way he gets a few drops each time—sugar water not enough for him." The nurse had a thought, but, to see if it was correct, asked the patient, "Do you think this is the only way the baby can get food until your milk comes in?" "Yes, it's all I got." The nurse knew that babies could have supplemental feedings and wondered what the patient thought about getting some. "Oh, yes, nurse, is better then, my baby will eat." Supplemental feedings were arranged. The patient put the baby to breast, but only at three-hour intervals because he took his formula eagerly after each nursing.

For a period of two days information about this patient was available, yet the behavior of the patient could not be modified. As soon as a nurse initiated a process of exploration of the matter with the patient, an understanding of the problem was reached, and its solution was worked out.

Examine briefly the comments the nurses and doctor exchanged about the patient. The persons involved formulated their comments probably as a consequence of direct experience with the patient. Interestingly enough, the comments which described what the patient was doing were correct, even from the patient's point of view. However, the thoughts and conclusions drawn were incorrect; they were arrived at independently and did not take into consideration how the patient might be regarding the problem. Instead, their own ideas were reflected in the comments. Had any of them told the patient what they thought, expressed their thoughts as questions, they might have enabled the patient to correct their mistaken conclusions. For example, the nurses might have said, "Don't you want any suggestions, because I'm concerned that your nipples will break down?" "Don't you understand that your milk isn't in yet?" or "Don't you want to listen to me?" In expressing their thoughts and exploring them with the patient, the nurses might have learned that the suggestions and concerns geared to protecting the mother's nipples were not those which would relieve the mother's concern about the baby's hunger, that the patient knew only too well that her milk wasn't in yet and that the patient heard the nurse, but wanted to give the baby what few drops of milk she had.

The activity the nurses engaged in with the patient should also be examined because the knowledge of this activity constituted available nursing data. One presumably explained that the patient's milk wasn't in yet; another directed the patient not to put the baby to breast every five minutes; another explained to the patient that her nipples would break down. Had any of them ascertained the effect of their activity on the patient, they might have learned that the patient already knew that her milk wasn't in yet, that she would continue to put the baby to breast every five minutes and that she didn't care if her nipples broke down. The nurses would then have realized that a service had not yet been provided for the patient.

Another outcome might also have been possible. Let us suppose the nurse explored the comments she heard at report but found out that the patient was not in distress. This might be so if, for example, the doctor on rounds *(while report was going on)* had identified the problem and ordered supplemental feedings. The nurse might not yet have been aware of the new order, but she would be obliged to find out that the information she had obtained was no longer useful. She may also have found out that what she heard at report was no longer relevant if she saw the new order and commented on it to the patient, "I notice the doctor ordered supplemental feedings. Do you know why he did?", etc. In this case, the patient would have been able to let her know that her problem had already been solved. The consideration of available and initially inadequate nursing data as they relate to the patient's need for help makes it possible to formulate the principle which guides the nurse in her practice of observation. *Any observation shared and explored with the patient is immediately useful in ascertaining and meeting his need or finding out that he is not in need at that time.*

What happened when the nurse did not apply this principle pointed up not only the importance of having done so but also the necessity to view the nurse-patient situation as a dynamic whole—how the patient behaves affects the nurse and the nurse in turn affects the patient. The interaction, or process which goes on between them, is unique for each situation.

ELEMENTS OF NURSING PROCESS

A nursing situation is comprised of three basic elements: (1) the behavior of the patient, (2) the reaction of the nurse, and (3) the nursing actions which are designed for the patient's benefit. The interaction of these elements with each other is nursing process. These elements will be examined here as each relates to the process of helping the patient and to the nurse's effective functioning.

The Patient's Behavior

The patient's behavior is behavior which is observed by the nurse in an immediate nurse-patient situation. For purposes of nursing it is possible to approach a description of behavior on the basis of what the nurse perceives. The word perception is used in a restricted sense, including only the stimuli the nurse experiences directly through her senses, *i.e., what she sees, what she touches, what she hears, what she smells, and what she tastes.*

The behavior of the patient may be perceived by the nurse in any of its following forms. Nonverbal expressions of behavior are manifest by motor activity *(e.g., eating, walking, twitching, trembling)* and physiological manifestations *(e.g., urinating, defecating, temperature and blood pressure readings, changes in respiration, skin color, etc.).* These forms are generally perceived visually. Essentially nonverbal behavior which is vocal may be heard by the nurse *(e.g., crying, moaning, laughing, coughing, wheezing, sighing, yelling, screaming, groaning, singing, etc.).* The verbal behavior of the patient which is perhaps more variable encompasses anything a patient says. It is possible to group all verbal behavior as complaints *(e.g., "I have pain." "I have a headache." "The food here is terrible." "I'm nervous." "I'm worried." "I'm afraid.");* requests *(e.g., "May I please have a glass of water?" "Please close the blinds for me." "May I have a bedpan?" "Will you call the doctor for me?" "Can I have something for my pain?");* questions *(e.g., "What school did you graduate from?" "Are you a new nurse?" "Am I going home?" "Are you short of nurses here?" "What does ambulatory mean?" "Should I tell the doctor when he comes?");* refusals *(e.g., "I'm sorry nurse but I can't do it." "I won't eat." "I don't want to drink." "I don't want that needle.");* demands *(e.g., "Get out of here!" "Get me a glass of water!" "If you don't do it, I'll sign myself out." "Give me a cigarette!" "I don't want to be disurbed!");* and any others as comments or statements *(e.g., "It's a nice day today." "Mrs. Smith, over there, didn't sleep all night.").* Verbal and nonverbal behavior can of course be observed simultaneously.

It is common for the nurse to perceive behavior in the patient's *"looks"* as shown by such comments as, "He looks so sad," "He looks miserable," and "He seems comfortable." Such statements are really thoughts which occur to the nurse as a consequence of perceiving some facet of behavior. For instance, the nurse may see the patient rubbing his abdomen and biting his lip, and therefore think the patient *"looks"* in pain. Other terms used to describe the *"looks"* of the patient might be: he *"looks"* tense, unhappy, worried, exhausted, uncomfortable, remote, glad, happy, angry, joyous, fearful, rigid, anxious, apprehensive, etc.

The following four illustrations point out how unimportant the patient's presenting behavior might seem and be of no professional concern until its meaning to the patient is understood.

A Patient "Looks" as if He Wants to Say Something

From a distance of approximately 10 feet a nurse saw a patient standing just inside the doorway of his room. Both his hands held the frame of the door as he bent forward looking out into the hall; his head turned right, then left. This behavior continued for about five minutes as the following ensued. A second nurse passed him on her way down the hall. His mouth opened, but he did not speak. The nurse smiled. The patient returned the smile. His head turned toward another nurse coming in the opposite direction. His mouth opened but closed again as the nurse passed. He resumed looking to the right, then to the left. A third nurse passed by and smiled. His mouth opened, but immediately closed, to smile as the third nurse continued walking and said, "So you're out of bed today. How nice." A fourth nurse approached the patient at the doorway with a medication tray and handed him a pill. He turned from the hallway into his room. The nurse poured some water and handed it to him. The nurse smiled, the patient's mouth opened, but he did not speak as the nurse left the room. He resumed his position and behavior at the doorway, but this time he was also scratching his face.

The nurse who had been watching him finally asked, "You look as though you want to say something. Do you?" The patient sighed deeply and immediately replied, "Oh, no, nurse—I need a robe. I have to go to the toilet quick, and I'm ashamed to walk down the hall in these pajamas."

A Patient "Looks" as if He's Exercising His Leg

Three times, a nurse saw a patient lifting his right leg up into the air and down again. Approximately half an hour later the nurse saw this identical behavior repeated. The nurse asked, "For the past half hour you look as though you've been exercising your leg. Have you?" The patient replied, gritting his teeth, "No, nurse, it just helps a little. I have a sharp pain in my back and it's killing me."

A Patient Requests Codeine for Pain

A patient spontaneously said to a nurse who had just entered her room, "Nurse, I would like to have codeine for my pain now." "Why do you want the codeine?" asked the nurse. "Because I'm uncomfortable." As the nurse explored the meaning of the pain and discomfort to the patient, the patient said, "It feels as though I have an abrasion on my thigh, and I simply can't stand that sticky, itchy sensation." Together they decided to clean away some old adhesive that was next to a new application. As the nurse did so the patient said, "Oh . . . that feels so good." When the nurse finished, a look of sheer pleasure crossed the patient's face as she said, "Boy, does this feel good. I had codeine two times last night and it didn't touch me. I don't need the codeine now."

A Patient Requests that the Nurse Fix Her Breast Binder

A patient spontaneously called out, "Nurse, would you kindly fix my breast binder?" This seemed incomprehensible to the nurse because the patient's binder was well pressed and looked fresh and appropriately applied. "Can you tell me why you want me to fix it?" The patient pulled her lips tight, bit the side of her cheek, hesitated, bit her lip and, as she started to cry said, "Because I'm having so much trouble. It isn't the binder, I just want to take very good care of my breasts. I'm so afraid that if I don't I won't be able to breast feed my baby."

In each of these illustrations, the *"looks"* or the requests were the patient's initial communications. They were not adequate to understand what the patients really meant or what they needed. However, exploration of the presenting behavior revealed the nature of their distress. On this basis the behavior which the nurse perceives must be viewed as a possible manifestation of an unmet need or a signal of distress. Admittedly, the nurse may discover that the patient does not require her help, but the patient's behavior must be viewed in this way in order to discover whether or not the patient is in need. For instance, a nurse may think the patient is in distress because she observes him limping along. When she investigates the patient may say, "I'm fine—nothing is the matter. I've had the limp all my life." Conversely the patient may seem comfortable to the nurse and not really be. An example is the retired university professor. When he started to ask his questions, he looked comfortable. Eventually the nurse found out that she was mistaken and that he clearly needed help. The nurse, therefore, assumes that the patient's behavior is a manifestation of distress or an unmet need unless, of course, she has evidence to the contrary. This does seem to be one way the nurse can maintain a correct awareness as to whether or not the patient requires her help at a given time.

The initial observations of the patient's presenting behavior are inadequate to understand what the patient is trying to communicate. Out of this phenomenon coupled with the patient's initial inability to communicate his needs emerges the principle which guides the nurse in her observations of the patient. *The presenting behavior of the patient, regardless of the form in which it appears, may represent a plea for help.*

The Nurse's Reaction

The second element of a nursing situation is the nurse's reaction. It consists of three aspects: *(1) perceptions of the patient's behavior, (2) the thoughts stimulated by the perceptions, and (3) feelings in response to these perceptions and thoughts.*

What the nurse perceives, thinks, and feels about the behavior of the patient will, of course, reflect her individuality, and will have more or less automatic consequences. Some nurses are more inclined to be aware of verbal forms of behavior before they notice nonverbal forms. Even when two nurses have the same perceptions, they may think and feel differently about them. For instance, both may see no mobility in the patient's eyes or face—one may think the patient is withdrawn and wish to help him; the other may think the patient is unfriendly and feel discomfort. Two nurses may hear a patient refuse a treatment—one may think the patient is upset and feel concern for him; the other may think the patient is uncooperative and feel frustrated. Although it is extremely difficult to separate perceptions from thoughts and feelings, it is worth trying to do so in order to focus attention on how one aspect of the nurse's reaction may affect the other aspects.

When the nurse perceives a patient, the thoughts which automatically occur to her reflect the meaning or interpretation she attaches to her perception. These meanings may or may not be correct from the patient's point of view. More than likely they are incorrect, or at least not completely correct, if we subscribe to the uniqueness of each person's experience. However, irrespective of their initial degree of accuracy, the perceptions which provoke the thoughts are communications from the patient. As a basis for discussing the individual nurse's reaction, the four examples cited in the discussion of patient behavior will be used.

The perceptions and thoughts of the two nurses about the patient who *"had to go to the toilet quick"* are notable for their individuality. One nurse noticed that the patient's mouth opened each time someone passed him, which made her think the patient wanted to say something. While she noticed the patient's mouth, the other nurse, seeing that the patient was out of bed, thought it was *"nice."* What the nurses saw and thought reflected their uniqueness in the experience with the patient.

One nurse perceived the motor activity of the patient's mouth and body. The other noted that the patient was out of bed. While the former perception seemed more relevant to the patient's distress, there was nothing wrong with the latter. What the individual nurse happens to perceive or think *(relevant or otherwise)* is not so important as what she does with it. What the nurse automatically perceives or thinks cannot ordinarily be controlled, but she can learn a responsive discipline, the discipline which phrases or formulates her perceptions or thoughts by questioning and wondering about the meaning of them to the patient. This kind of exploration enables the patient, in turn, to respond by expressing the meaning the nurse's perception or thought has to him. The story of the man who *"had to go to the toilet quick"* illustrates this point.

The nurse who said to the patient that it was nice to see him out of bed did not invite him to communicate how differently he felt at the same moment. Had she, her comments might have gone like this, "It's nice to see you out of bed now; how is it for you?" Although the second nurse did not tell the patient she saw his mouth open each time someone passed him, she did express that she thought he wanted to say something. She invited the patient to respond by asking if her thought was correct.

An invitation is implicit in questions which specifically explore the behavior the nurse recognizes or has a thought about. In the examples of the two patients who made requests and of the patient who looked as if he were exercising his leg, each patient immediately responded to the nurse's exploration by stating the meaning of the behavior the nurse was reacting to. Sometimes the patient may not answer the nurse when she explores his behavior. However, the absence of a verbal response is a form of nonverbal behavior which may also be explored. The nurse might ask, "Is there some reason why you cannot answer me?" The patient for one reason or another may still not feel safe enough to disclose what is on his mind. This barrier to their communication would have to be resolved before the nurse can be of help. The patient may be reacting against the nurse, the hospital, the doctor or another nurse, and may not yet be quite sure that his reaction will really be understood. In instances such as these, the patient may require additional demonstration of the nurse's interest. These assurances seem to work better when they are stated in the negative, *e.g.,* *"Is it that you don't think I'll understand?" "Am I wrong?" "I know you respect your doctor, but did he say something that you don't quite agree with . . . ?" "It looked like that procedure was very painful, and you didn't say a word about it."* The interesting thing about this is that, when the nurse raises possibilities with negative connotations, the patient experiences the permission and responds with his own *"negative"* reaction. Excerpts of a case example may illustrate this point.

A Patient's Face Flushes

A truck driver "who had never been sick a day in his life" was admitted as an emergency following a near fatal accident. In talking to the nurse several months later, the patient told her that, while he was in the emergency room, the doctors looked as if they had little hope for him. He was hemorrhaging, his bowel and bladder had ruptured, and he had multiple fractures of the bones below the waist. He had grabbed the doctor's arm and said, "Please, please, please, save my life."

The patient was in the hospital for eight months during which time several operations were performed. His response to treatment and his healing progressed rapidly. He respected and loved all the doctors and nurses who helped him, and, as he once expressed it, "If I lived 10 lifetimes, I could never thank them enough. They saved my life, they did for me what God couldn't do."

One morning the patient said, "Thank you," to a nurse who delivered his breakfast tray. His face became exceedingly red as he started to eat. Another nurse stopped and said, "You look as though you are going to eat those cold greasy eggs." "Yes, they are all right; they are like this whenever we have them." "Would you like me to fry you some that will at least look better than those?" "Oh, no, please don't bother. It's too much trouble." "If your only reason is that you don't want to trouble me, you're wrong. It will be no trouble." "You mean you really would . . . you mean I can really have decent fried eggs after all these months?" The nurse was about to leave as the patient said, "While you're at it, make me some toast that won't break my teeth."

The nurse returned with hot eggs and toast. As the patient ate, he said "You know—there have been days when I felt like throwing the tray at whoever brought it. If my wife ever served me food like that, I'd beat her within an inch of her life." "Why have you been so reluctant to tell people about how you wanted your food?" "You just can't, because everybody here is really wonderful. They might misunderstand my complaints and I wouldn't want them to think for a second that I'm ungrateful." The patient paused, smiled, squinted, then said, "You know, come to think of it, I haven't blown my top for eight months— it's funny, I just realized it and I used to—nearly every day."

The perception of the nurse is more often than not correct. It is unlikely that the patient would deny the statement of it if he is aware of the stimulus at the moment the event transpires. The patients discussed previously would not have, for example, denied being out of bed, requesting codeine, requesting that the nurse fix the breast binder, bringing the leg up in the air and down again. On the other hand, the patient whose face became red may have had an angry feeling but could not see his face flushing and therefore may have denied that his face was red. However, the individual and automatic thought the nurse has about her perception is likely to be inadequate or not completely correct unless it is first investigated with the patient. Indeed, thoughts are sometimes completely incorrect. The illustrations point out that when the nurse expressed her thought and asked the patient about it, the patient not only corrected her, but volunteered the specific meaning of the behavior she perceived. For instance, when the nurse asked the patient if he wanted to say something, he replied, "Oh, no, nurse, I need a robe quick." When the nurse asked if the patient was exercising his leg, he said, "No, nurse, it just helps a little." Thus, the nurse's automatic thoughts were misinterpretations or inadequate interpretations of why the patients behaved as they did. One patient exercised his leg, not for the sake of exercise, but for the purpose of helping his pain a little. Hence, the nurse may not take it for granted what the patient's behavior means to him.

In regard to the two patients who made requests, it is interesting to note that the nurse brought more immediate clarification into the situations when she questioned only what she heard them request: "Why codeine?" "Why fix the breast binder?" Without having to correct the nurse, the patients supplied the specific meaning of what the nurse perceived. Thus, ascertaining the meaning of behavior perhaps takes less time when the nurse explores only what she perceives, *e.g., "I notice you open your mouth every time someone passes. Can you tell me why?" "Can you tell me why you are bringing your leg up into the air and down again?" "Why do you want codeine?" "Can you tell me why you want me to fix your breast binder?"*

However, thoughts do occur automatically, and when expressed tentatively, even though they are incorrect or inadequate, they convey the permission which helps the patient express his own meaning. This happened when the nurses expressed what they thought their perceptions meant: "You look as though you've been exercising your leg. Have you?" "You look as though you want to say something. Do you?" Both patients were then immediately able to correct the nurses by answering "no" and adding their own meanings. A nurse's ability to hold her thoughts in abeyance might therefore not seem too important, and perhaps it is not. However, in more complicated processes, the amount of time involved in ascertaining the specific meaning of the patient's communications may become a problem. A patient may be in serious distress and the nurse may waste much time in exploring thoughts as they occur to her, only to find each time that they are incorrect. Therefore, it might be suggested that the nurse explore perceptions first, provided she has developed sufficient skill to do so or a responsive discipline as a result of experience, reconstruction and reflection. Automatic thoughts which do occur and how nurses can best use them are the present concern.

The stimulus the nurse reacts to may be something in the patient's immediate environment rather than his behavior. These reactions may also serve a useful purpose even if the stimulus which provokes them seems at the onset to be irrelevant to the patient's need for help. For example, a nurse with a very heavy assignment entered a patient's room. The patient was looking out the window. Neither looked at the other. The nurse stopped short and stared at the bed, which was freshly made, then said out loud, "What a surprise! Has someone taken care of you so soon?" The patient's head turned from the window as she said, "No, nurse, they just made my bed. I need a clean gown and towel so I can go wash myself."

In perceiving that the bed was made, the nurse thought the patient had been cared for. Because she explored her surprise, she became aware of the patient's need.

At this point in the discussion of the nurse's reaction, it may be concluded that the nurse's attempt to explore her perceptions or thoughts about the patient's behavior is crucial in understanding more fully what the patient is trying to communicate to her. The next point for consideration is: Why is it so important for the nurse to find out the meaning to the patient of her reaction in the immediate situation?

Nurses may often hear such expressions as, "Let well enough alone." "Don't bring it up." "Don't be so direct." "Wait for the patient to take the initiative before you discuss something." "Don't tell the patient; see what happens." Directives such as these deny or avoid what may actually be taking place. When the reaction of the nurse, in any of its aspects, is not explored with the patient, his condition remains unchanged or becomes worse. This of course presupposes that the patient's need has not been met.

Nurses Hear a Patient Scream

At morning report the night nurse said, "Mrs. C. came in 24 hours ago. You probably know her." Another nurse replied, "Do I? She screamed all evening—even paraldehyde didn't stop her for a minute." The night nurse added, "She kept it up all night— like she's screaming now, and all the patients on the ward have been awake most of the night."

The patient was still screaming as a nurse reviewed the nurse's notes and read: "9 A.M.—admitted, moaning and mumbling, restraints applied, side rails on bed." "5 P.M.—disoriented, screaming." "7:15 P.M.—culture, stool and urine sent to lab, screamed all evening, paraldehyde 15 cc."; "11:30 P.M.—very disoriented." "12 midnight—very noisy and confused, screaming, incontinent, paraldehyde 15 cc."; "2 A.M.—very noisy, screaming at the top of her voice, disoriented, paraldehyde 15 cc."; "6 A.M.—screaming constantly, paraldehyde 15 cc."

The patient was still screaming when the nurse entered her room. While the patient screamed, the nurse said, "I came in because you're screaming. Can you tell me what's wrong?" The patient stopped screaming and said, "Yes, I certainly can tell you. I want to turn on my back—my side is killing me."

When the patient was turned, the nurse asked, "How does it feel now?" "Better," said the patient, "but I still have a lot of pain. I haven't slept for 24 hours, and I am tired." Without clearly discerning what the patient now needed, the nurse decided to get medication for pain and asked the patient if it was all right for her to do so. The patient said, "Well, of course." In leaving, the nurse asked if the patient was able to use the call light in the event that she needed the nurse before her return. The patient lifted her head, picked up the bell, and said, "Will you come? They don't, you know, no matter how hard I scream." The nurse said that she would. The patient smiled, dropped the cord light and the nurse left. Three minutes later the nurse returned to tell the patient she had not yet received an order for medication, but found the patient asleep, holding the bell cord with both hands.

Over a period of 16 hours nurses heard a patient scream, but they did not use this perception to understand how to go about helping her. The nurse who did initiate exploration of the screaming found out its immediate meaning to the patient.

All the nurses probably had the same perception *(screaming)*, but the validity of perceptions does not necessarily depend on their agreement with those of other nurses. At different times nurses may perceive different behavior because the behavior of the patient has actually changed. Even though different aspects of seemingly different behavior are perceived, the unmet need giving rise to it remains the same. Moreover, it appears that the longer the patient is frustrated in getting help, the more distressful the presenting behavior becomes and the more obscure its meaning. For example, the perception of the night nurse who heard Mrs. Smith complain about going to the bathroom too often, did not agree with the day nurse's perception when the patient complained of pain. These perceptions were different, but were expressions of the same distress. *"Pain"* would ordinarily be thought of as a more distressful complaint than *"going to the bathroom too often."* Certainly, the distress of the patient who was screaming became progressively more intense from the time she was admitted, as indicated in the nurses' notes and from her moaning and mumbling which progressed to screaming that became louder and louder. It seems as though the patient tries to communicate his distress first in one way, and, as it increases, in another way. Naturally, the nurses who administered paraldehyde thought it would help the screaming. As stated previously, thoughts are always a useful point of departure for exploration, if the patient is invited to respond. The thought that "paraldehyde will help the patient's screaming" might have been expressed as, "The doctor left an order for some medicine which I think will help. Do you?" This suggestion might appear too naive to consider. However, exploring thoughts such as these will be discussed in subsequent material. We do know that the nurse who heard screaming and thought something was wrong did explore her reaction and was able to help the patient. Also, until the nurse did conduct the inquiry, the patient's behavior became progressively more distressed.

Sometimes the nurse may state a thought in such a way as to make it hard for the patient to explain his distress. This may happen even though the thought is expressed as a question. For example:

A Patient "Looks" as if He Is in Pain

A nurse was performing tasks in rapid succession. Suddenly she stopped short at a bedside only to nod and say, "You are all right, aren't you?" The patient replied, "Yes, nurse." The nurse picked up linen and an I.V. pole and rushed out of the room. Another nurse immediately approached the same patient and said, "That nurse just asked if you were all right. You said you were, but you don't seem all right to me. Am I wrong?" "No, you're right. It's the pain in my leg, nurse; it's really very bad and I don't think I'm going to be able to stand it much longer."

The nurse who helped the patient verbalize his complaint wanted to find out the perception and true thoughts of the nurse who asked the patient if he was all right. She asked, "Why did you ask the patient if he was all right?" The first nurse replied, "Because he looked as if he was in pain. Even though he said he was all right I didn't think so but I couldn't stop because the doctor was waiting for the I.V. pole."

Thus, a thought expressed as a question may not help the patient verbalize his discomfort unless he feels the nurse wants to hear about it. Moreover, the first nurse did not really express or explore her true perception or thoughts with the patient. What she did express was almost a wish for reassurance that he was all right because she was preoccupied and in the midst of rapidly reacting to another task.

So far, we have only highlighted the perceptive and thinking aspects of the nurse's reaction and have made almost no reference to feelings *per se*. Ordinarily, and prior to learning how to deliberate on the process of her reaction, the nurse's perceptions, thoughts and feelings are experienced almost simultaneously. She perceives, has automatic thoughts about her perceptions *(if her thoughts are not tentatively formulated as questions and wonderings, she assumes they are correct)*, and then she feels a certain way.

Concern, interest, liking, and desire to help are examples of appropriate feelings. Undesirable feelings with a negative connotation include anger, fury, dislike, annoyance, and impatience. Whether or not the feeling is a desirable one, it may lead to results which may help or harm the patient, depending on the validity of the thoughts preceding the feeling and what the nurse does with it. A positive or negative feeling may function as usefully as perceptions and thoughts, provided it is explored in such a way that the patient is invited to react to it. In this way, the nurse is able to ascertain the difference or similarity between her feeling and the patient's. By questioning the patient about her feeling, she finds out if it is or is not helpful to the patient at that time. Interestingly enough, even positive feelings often go unresolved, as illustrated by the nurse who did not express and explore her concern about the patient's nipples breaking down. She might have stated it as, "I'm concerned that your nipples will break down. Why aren't you?" This question might have helped the patient tell the nurse that her baby's hunger was more important at the moment.

If the nurse does not resolve her feeling with the patient in the situation, she may see the patient later on and have the same feeling again without ever finding out its usefulness to the patient, thus seeming to reinforce it. In addition, if the feeling is not expressed and explored, it may show in the nurses' nonverbal behavior, *i.e., by the way she looks, by her tone, or by the way she moves or handles equipment or touches the patient's body.* Nonverbal manifestations of anger, impatience, concern and liking are often readily apparent. The nurse who does not tell the patient what her feelings are allows him to interpret the nonverbal manifestation of them in his own way. Thus, the real problem in relation to the nurse's feelings appears to be that they are not automatically understood by the patient. The important point is not whether the nurse's feeling is positive or negative, but were the thoughts provoking the feeling correct and how does her feeling affect the patient. Moreover, the evaluation of a feeling as positive or negative depends on the person who has it or on the person who is being affected by it.

The following four illustrations show how feelings may come about automatically and point out that (1) even if feelings are positive but derived from thoughts which are not first checked with the patient, they do not benefit him, and (2) the patient can make use of the nurse's feeling when she expresses it, *provided she explains the basis for it and allows the patient to correct or validate what her feeling is about.*

A Patient Commands: The Nurse Feels Angry

The behavior of Mrs. Crane, for several weeks, was such that the nurses found it difficult to like her. One of the nurses said to another, "You'd think she'd start treating us better, since we obey her every command. She's impossible, and that's all there is to it."

The next day, another nurse reluctantly entered Mrs. Crane's room. She had been avoiding the patient except for answering the call light. She disliked being ordered around because she knew she could do what the patient wanted without emphatic orders.

"Come get me off this bedpan!" said the patient whose legs were paralyzed. The nurse automatically felt as angry as she had on previous occasions but did not express her anger. Instead, she sighed deeply and said, "All right." The nurse already had toilet tissue in her hand when the patient said, "You get the paper! Give me some. I'll wipe here—you wipe there." Before the nurse started to wipe the area that the patient had directed, the patient said, "Do better. It's not dry—clean better!" The more demands the patient issued, the angrier the nurse became, because she thought she was perfectly capable of wiping the patient without having to be ordered around. "You know, the more you tell me what to do the angrier I become. It's as though you think I don't know anything. Is that why you continually give orders?"

The patient reached out her hand, tears filled her eyes, her mouth quivered as she sighed, then said, "Close the door so no one will hear me. I will tell you the secrets of my soul."

The patient's secrets had to do with how fearful she was of her back "breaking down." She told the nurse she had been paralyzed for three years, and during the first year she "died with pain from bedsores. . . . When the nurses are busy—they don't wipe well and the urine goes to my back. I have to be careful and tell the nurses how to take care of me."

The nurse said thoughtfully, "So far then your telling the nurses what to do has prevented a bed sore? Can I tell the other nurses, because I don't think they know? I didn't, and

I'm sure they don't want your back to break down either."
"Yes, nurse, you're so good, you give me courage to walk."

The patient's demanding behavior stopped. The nurse who thought Mrs. Crane was impossible had occasion to see her the next day. After she left the patient's room, she said, "It's incredible. I can't believe it. Mrs. Crane is a different person."

Undoubtedly the patient's distress and the nurse's anger would have become more and more intense if the nurse had not explored how she felt with the patient. It is important to note that the nurse's anger was a direct outcome of her incorrect idea about why the patient was ordering her around. However, in expressing her anger, the basis for it, and by inviting the patient to respond, the nurse was able to correct her thoughts and her angry feeling. It was easy for the nurse to feel concern instead of anger but only after she understood the meaning of the demands to the patient. What the patient was trying to achieve was commendable from any nurse's point of view.

Although the primary interest is in preventing angry and undesirable feelings as well as retaliatory reactions to the patient, it must be recognized that the nurse like any other person may develop feelings which do not help the patient, despite her best efforts. But, despite her feelings, the nurse is still responsible for caring for her patients. The way the nurse resolved her anger in the previous illustration was not only beneficial to the patient, but also helped the nurse to function more effectively. In using the method which is suggested here, the nurse, in expressing her feeling, must be sure to explain the thoughts which provoked it and invite the patient to react to it. It was important for the nurse to explain the basis of her feeling to Mrs. Crane. Otherwise, the patient would have learned only that the nurse was angry which would have meant to the patient, *The nurse is angry just because I want to make sure my back doesn't break down.*

A Patient Makes a Request: The Nurse Feels Furious

A patient asked, "Would you do me a favor nurse?" The nurse nodded as the patient said, "Call this number and ask for my sister Dorothy. When she answers tell her I want her to come and see me today." The nurse did not explore the meaning of this request to the patient. The nurse dialed the number but got no answer. The patient gave the nurse another number. Dorothy was not there. As the nurse waited for a dial tone for the seventh time, she said to another nurse, "Calling all these numbers is ridiculous and unnecessary, and I'm furious because I'm beginning to feel like a telephone operator." The nurse was sighing heavily and her face was red. The other nurse said, "Have you told the patient what's happening or asked her why she's doing this to you?" "No, but I will now." Returning to the patient she said, "This is getting ridiculous, and I'm furious. I don't think it's necessary for me to make useless telephone calls. I'm beginning to feel like a tele-phone operator. What's this message I have to give all about?" "Oh, I'm sorry, nurse, but it's very important. I've been trying to reach my sister for three days now. She's minding my children— she said she'd come to see me but I don't know what has hap-pened. I just want to make sure the children are all right."

The nurse's face was no longer red as she said, "I'm sorry too. No wonder you are thinking up every number in the book, although I do think it will be better if we ask the police to find her. Is that all right with you?" "Oh, yes, nurse, that would be better because I don't know who to call next."

When the nurse expressed what she thought and felt and why, and invited the patient to respond, the patient explained the basis for her request. The explanation changed the nurse's angry feeling to one of concern—a feeling more consistent with the patient's need.

Early in the interaction the nurse started to think that the telephone calls were unnecessary. Had she not assumed that this thought was correct and explored it instead then she would not have become furious. She would have been as concerned as she was near the conclusion of the interaction.

In the following situation a nurse developed a positive feel-ing which led to a result which did not help the patient.

A Patient "Looks" Startled: A Nurse Assumes He Is
Confused and Feels Concern

Two days previously, a patient had been transferred from a locked to an open ward. On this particular day he was walking down the hall when the head nurse said to him, "Your dental appointment is at 10 A.M." The patient looked startled but he did not speak, blinked his eyes and then squinted. The head nurse asked, "What's the matter?" but did not pursue her questioning and allowed the patient to walk away. At 10:30 A.M. the dental clinic notified the nurse that the patient had not kept his appointment. At 3:00 P.M., when the patient returned, the head nurse asked, "Where have you been?" The patient did not answer. Later the nurse said to the doctor, "This patient is very confused today, and I'm really concerned about him. He left the ward at 9:45 A.M. to go to the dental clinic, but he didn't get there. He wouldn't tell me where he had been when he returned at 3:00 P.M. I'm not sure it's safe to keep him on the open ward."

Arrangements were made for the patient to be transferred back to the locked ward. When the patient arrived, he said to the nurse whom he knew, "I don't belong here, I was getting better." "Can you tell me why you think you don't belong?" The patient did not answer. The nurse then said, "Since I don't know why you think you don't belong, I'll tell you what I know. They were concerned about you because they thought you were confused again. You left the ward for the dentist's office but you got lost somewhere, and, to be sure you are protected, they transferred you here. Does any of this make sense to you?" "It makes sense, but I didn't get lost and I wasn't confused. I was scared—afraid of that *damn* drilling! I was shaking all over and I just couldn't get up nerve enough to go. I sat in the corner of the coffee shop for hours hoping I'd find the courage to go. Finally, about 2:30, I felt better and went to the clinic, but they couldn't take me. They told me they would make another appointment."

The head nurse's positive feeling of concern for the patient's safety was based on her incorrect thought from observation of the patient, a conclusion she assumed was correct but which was based on insufficient data. The fact that the patient did not answer her questions and did not keep his appointment did not mean that he was confused. As soon as the basis of concern was explored with the patient, he was able to clarify the meaning of what had been observed. Had the head nurse pursued her exploration of the patient's behavior at the onset and learned that the patient was scared, she may still have felt concern, but a different nursing action would have been decided upon. Thus, a positive feeling unexpressed and not explored with the patient did not benefit him. The patient's distress became known when the feeling of concern and its basis were explained, and he in turn was invited to respond with his own meaning.

A Patient Refuses to Eat

A Nurse Feels *"Awful but Concerned"*

A Nurses Aide Feels *"Sick and Tired"*

The patient was 60 years of age. His leg had been amputated during a previous admission and his right arm during the current admission. At mealtimes, personnel who knew him would stop at the door and ask, "Are you going to eat?" The patient would not answer, and the tray would be returned to the kitchen. Those who did not know the patient would enter and attempt to place his tray. In response the patient would yell, "You s _____ of a b_____, get it out of here." He would also attempt to throw the dishes on the floor. This behavior continued for three days. Daily intravenous solutions were ordered and during their administration the patient had to be restrained.

The nurse who made the above observations felt concern but did not express it or the basis for it. Instead, she explored the patient's refusal to eat. Just before an intravenous was to be administered, she tried to find out how to help him, "As far as I know, you are capable of eating, but why won't you?" "Because I want to die." When she asked the patient why, she discovered that the only people he knew or who cared about him, his wife and his son, were dead. He said that he had no reason to live and that, even if he did, he couldn't work with only one arm and one leg. Although the nurse felt sorry for the patient she didn't think he should starve himself to death but failed to express it. Instead, she said, "Your breakfast is here and if you don't like what's on it, I'll get whatever I can that you do like. I

just feel awful when they restrain you for the intravenous."
"Listen, you are a nice nurse, but you don't understand. I have
no reason to live. I want to die. Don't you understand that?" The
nurse felt overwhelmed and left the room.

In the utility room the nurse initiated a discussion about the
patient with the nurse's aide who generally prepared the equipment for the intravenous. The aide banged the tray that was in
his hand and said, "I'm sick and tired of his refusing to eat. I'm
going to try to make him eat by shoving it down his throat.
That's the only way. If he throws the tray at me, I'll give up and
get the intravenous ready."

The nurse followed the aide as he walked into the room with
the breakfast tray, saying, "I'm sick and tired of your not eating.
If you want to die, I'm not going to help you do it. Here! Unless
you throw the tray at me, you are going to eat." As he said,
"here" he held the patient's nose and forced him to swallow.
The patient did not fight—a dramatic change in his response to
food. The patient allowed the aide to feed him, so that it was not
necessary to hold his nose again. When the aide left, the nurse
asked, "Why is it you didn't fight the aide as you did others
who have asked you to eat?" "Because he's the only one who
really cares whether I live or die—he made me eat." The patient resumed eating three meals a day.

The nurse was concerned about the patient, but did not
make her concern and the reason for it explicit. Later, when
she told the patient she felt awful when they restrained him for
the intravenous, she did not invite the patient to tell her how
he felt about it. In addition, she did not persist in exploring her
thoughts in order to find out what the patient specifically
required of her. On the other hand, even though we may question the aide's method of meeting the patient's need *(a force-
ful demonstration to make him eat),* the aide did adhere to the
conditions which make it possible for the patient to benefit
from reactions to him. The aide expressed the way he felt; the
basis for it; and invited the patient to react. The patient responded to the limited invitation by passively permitting the
aide to feed him. The nurse's approach seemed to be more

appropriate but it was the way the aide used his reaction that helped the patient.

In situations like the one just cited, patients may not respond verbally when the nurse explores her reaction. The nurse may have no other recourse but to test out her thoughts and feelings in action and watch for results in the nonverbal behavior, *e.g., when the aide expressed his reaction and acted it out, the patient did not answer, but responded nonverbally.* He became passive in the face of the aide's determination—a marked contrast to the strong resistance of which he was capable.

The illustrations thus far point out that any aspect of the nurse's reaction, perception, thought or feeling expressed and explored enables the patient to communicate the information the nurse needs in order to be of help. When the nurse does not explore with the patient her reaction *(expressed or unexpressed),* it seems reasonably certain that clear communication between them stops. If exploration of the perceptions does not work, the nurse can explore the thoughts which occur to her. But if this does not work, she can explore her feelings and the basis for them. It seems to make little difference which aspect of the reaction she chooses to inquire about first. Choosing what is uppermost in her own mind at any given moment is probably as valid as any other criterion for selection. That she resolve the reaction is her professional concern not only to benefit the patient but to foster her work satisfaction as well.

It is now possible to formulate a principle to guide the nurse in her process of reacting to the patient. *The nurse does not assume that any aspect of her reaction to the patient is correct, helpful or appropriate until she checks the validity of it in exploration with the patient.*

A nurse may undergo other reactions which may negatively influence the nurse-patient situation. These reactions arise from responses to the setting which have little to do with the individual patient for whom she is then caring. These reactions will be discussed only briefly in the belief that they may be either avoided, easily resolved, or unproblematic, if the nurse is clear about her professional role and identity.

Reactions which the nurse does not resolve may interfere with the interaction between herself and a patient. These reactions may stem from her personal or professional frame of reference, *i.e., her personal codes of behavior, her personal value system or her own ideas as to what a nurse should or should not do and say.* More immediately her reactions may be stimulated by the patient or may result from interaction with other people such as another patient, the head nurse, supervisor or doctor. Any reactions with which the nurse remains preoccupied impedes the process of helping the patient usually because they have not been expressed and explored in the situation which provoked them. In such instances it can be assumed that the nurse has not yet learned how useful exploration of her reactions may be. She has not yet *"earned"* the professional security which comes about when her personal reactions are explored for their professional references and validity. Instead of responding in terms of her actual experience, she responds in terms of what she automatically assumes is expected of her. Two such reactions will be illustrated. In both, it can be noted that the process of reacting and the problems which ensue are similar to those which occur between a patient and a nurse. With both persons involved there is automatic action and reaction without mutual understanding and without recognition of the need to initiate a process of resolution.

A Patient Tells a Nurse the Same Story Ten Times

One nurse was telling another, "That patient keeps telling the same story over and over again. I've heard it 10 times and if I hear it again, I'll scream." The other nurse said, "I couldn't listen to the same story 10 times unless there was a special reason. Did you ask him why he keeps telling you the same story?" "I wouldn't dare." "Why not?" "Well, because I should listen and accept him; he can't help it if he's mentally ill,—besides, I don't want to be impolite."

The next time the patient repeated the story, the nurse explored her reaction by saying, "I don't want to sound impolite, but I can't help wondering why you keep telling me the same story over and over again." The patient replied, "Well, that's a relief. You looked as if you were listening, but I wasn't really sure. I just wanted to be sure you knew how miserable that woman made my life."

The patient told a story ten times. Although the nurse reacted, she did not express or explore it for reasons having to do with politeness and what she thought was the *"right"* behavior of a nurse—neither of which was helpful to the patient. Until such time as she expressed and explored her reaction, she couldn't understand why the patient behaved as he did nor could the patient know in any real way that she was listening to what he had to say.

A Head Nurse Issues a Directive

It was 10 A.M. A new nurse on the unit was about to finish caring for a patient. The patient had been awake all night. She felt *"too sick"* to eat breakfast, but, since her needs had been ascertained and met, she was feeling better. In addition, she now said she was hungry. The nurse supplied milk and crackers. As the patient wiped her lips, she said, "That milk was good. You are a real angel of mercy. I'm about to fall asleep like nobody in this hospital ever slept before. Now don't forget, you promised to keep a watch out for me so nobody wakes me—that is, until supper." The nurse made arrangements not to waken the patient for lunch, and saved fruit and milk in the event the patient awoke and became hungry before the evening meal.

At 12:15 the head nurse approached and said, "Listen, your patient's twelve o'clock temperature isn't recorded yet. Take it and record it as soon as you can. The doctors will be on rounds any minute now because they didn't come this morning, and, if Dr. X. sees a temperature not taken, he'll blow his top." The nurse hesitated but then nodded, went to the patient's room and awakened the patient. The patient said, "Oh, no—and you promised I could sleep. What do they want with my temperature? I don't have any fever." The nurse said, "I'm terribly sorry, but the doctor wants it now and I have to take it." The patient said, "It's okay, I know it's not your fault."

In the utility room the same nurse initiated a discussion with another by saying, "What's the use? Even when you have the time to give a patient good care, you can't. A stupid temperature is more important than what the patient needs? As far as I can see, there was no reason to take it. I promised her I'd let her sleep, but the head nurse told me to take the temperature, and, of course, it was normal."

"Were you reasonably certain that she had no elevation?" "Well, as sure as I could be without actually taking it. She didn't have an elevation at 8:00 A.M. and was very comfortable before she fell asleep." "What you say makes sense, but why was it that you didn't tell the head nurse?" "Well, I suppose I could have, and I was going to, but she said Dr. X. would blow his top if he found it was not recorded."

Clearly there was nothing *"wrong"* with the head nurse's directive to have the staff nurse record a routine temperature, as this is another way nurses *"watch out"* for patients. Automatically, the head nurse thought of Dr. X. when she found it had not been recorded. It is not unlikely that someone had once omitted an important recording of temperature, and for that reason Dr. X. *"blew his top."* It is most unlikely that he would react that way if the situation had been explained to him. However, neither the doctor nor the head nurse had the information which would have made an omission of a temperature helpful to the patient. Yet, when the head nurse directed the staff nurse to take the temperature as soon as she could, the nurse automatically thought it was *"stupid,"* but went right ahead and assumed that the temperature was more important to the head nurse and the doctor than the patient's need.

Nothing was *"wrong"* with the nurse's reaction. Her reasoning and conclusions were based on the real data she had about the patient. It was almost as if she expected the head nurse to know automatically that taking the temperature would disturb the patient. What did go wrong was that the nurse did not express and explore her reaction with the head nurse. Had she, the problem in caring for the patient might have been avoided. It was not possible for the head nurse to make a more appropriate decision without the opportunity to do so. It might even be said that the head nurse could not make any other decision without having first received additional information from the staff nurse.

In a way, the nurse who automatically complied with the directive had not yet learned how to deal with the legitimate authority of the head nurse so that her effective work with the patient could continue without unnecessary restraint.

In turn, if the head nurse had the necessary information and decided that the patient should be allowed to sleep, she may or may not have been able to deal with Dr. X. She would have been faced with two possibilities. The doctor would have either agreed with the reason for the omission or he may have insisted on having the temperature taken. The nurse would then have had to find out why the temperature was to take precedence over the patient's need for sleep. For example, the nurse may have found out that the reading was essential for an accurate diagnosis and was the reason why the patient was being hospitalized *(at a cost to the patient of $28 per day)*. If this were the case, the nurse would not have objected to waking the patient nor would the patient have objected either. On the other hand, the nurse might have been unsuccessful in finding out why the temperature reading was more important than the patient's need for sleep. In such an instance, she can be reasonably certain that she had not yet understood the basis for the doctor's judgment or that she had not yet given the doctor sufficient information for him to understand the basis for her own. In either case, further discussion would be necessary. A similar line of reasoning and method of procedure is indicated with whomever else the nurse deals in caring for her patients.

The nurse's unresolved reactions to people other than her patients may, therefore, interfere with her function. These reactions may seem positive or negative depending on the person who is judging them. If the nurse is preoccupied with either, she is less available to the patient for whom she is caring. If she is reacting against some other person, she is less able to respond to her patient with warmth and interest. Even extraneous positive reactions may interfere with the process of helping a patient, *e.g., when the nurse automatically complies and willingly carries out requests, directives, orders, etc.,* while her patients are needing something different. On this basis, we might emphasize that the nurse is responsible to resolve extraneous reactions, positive or negative, which interfere with helping patients. She is professionally obligated to initiate the resolution of them.

The Nurse's Activity

The third element of a nursing situation consists of any action the nurse carries out. It includes only what she says or does with or for the benefit of the patient. These actions may be decided upon with or without the patient's participation and are essentially of two types: *(1) actions decided upon deliberatively—those which ascertain or meet the patient's immediate need—and (2) automatic activities—those decided upon for reasons other than the patient's immediate need.* Some automatic activities are ordered by the doctor; others are concerned with routines of caring for patients, and still others are based on principles pertinent to protecting and fostering the health of people in general.

Although some actions are decided upon independently of the patient, it must be emphasized that they are designed for the purpose of helping him. The nurse may carry out actions which are deliberative or automatic by *instructing, suggesting, directing, explaining, informing, requesting, questioning, making decisions for the patient, by handling the body of the patient, administering medications or treatments* or by *changing the patient's immediate environment.*

While it is evident that routines of care, medical orders and activities based on health principles, are designed for the purpose of helping the patient, deliberation is needed to determine whether the activity actually achieves its intended purpose and whether the patient is helped by it.

A distinction needs to be made here between the purpose an activity actually serves and its intended purpose of helping the patient. For instance, if a nurse decides to make a bed for the purpose of having it made, her activity achieves purpose, but it may not help the patient. The case report of the patient who screamed continuously illustrates this point: if the nurses who administered paraldehyde did so for the purpose of carrying out a doctor's order, then it follows that the purpose of that activity was achieved. However, the activity did not achieve its intended purpose—to reduce or stop the screaming and thereby help the patient.

What a nurse says or does is necessarily an outcome of her reaction to something in the situation. Specific perceptions, thoughts or feelings precipitate her action. Thoughts and feelings in direct response to perceptions of the patient's behavior were discussed earlier. Sometimes, although the nurse perceives the patient's behavior, she may automatically think of doctors' orders, policies, routines, health principles and so on. Automatic thoughts such as these are not really relevant to the meaning of a patient's behavior but may be the professional concern of the nurse. For instance, some nurses heard a patient screaming and presumably thought of the doctor's order, or that paraldehyde helps to quiet patients, or assumed that paraldehyde was indicated and decided to give it. The purpose of administering it was to relieve the condition which caused the screaming, but although paraldehyde was administered, the screaming continued. The activity did not achieve its purpose nor did it help the patient.

Thus, if a nurse automatically acts on any perception, thought or feeling without exploring it further with the patient, the activity may very well be ineffective in achieving its purpose or in helping the patient. On the other hand, if the nurse checks her thoughts and explores her reactions with the patient before deciding on which action to follow, what she does is more likely to achieve its purpose and help the patient. Another nurse who heard the same patient screaming checked with the patient before she decided what to do. The patient needed a change in position. When her need was met she stopped screaming and slept.

It is desirable, of course, for the nurse to keep in mind doctors' orders, health principles, policies, and so on, and it is understandable when she thinks of these things in response to her perceptions of the patient. Automatic thoughts such as these explored with a patient can serve as usefully as those which explore the meaning of a patient's behavior. This point will be illustrated in the next case example. In spite of the importance of checking with the patient before acting, actions may take place as quickly and as automatically as thoughts before discussion with the patient. If the nurse does not conduct the inquiry before she acts, she may do so while she acts or after the activity is completed. It does seem that time is saved if she inquires before acting. Whether the nurse tries to find out what is happening to the patient before, during, or after the activity, she should permit the patient to react; in order to know how the patient anticipates, experiences or is affected by the activity.

The specific conditions which affect the process of the nurse's activity in helping the patient will now be identified in order to establish guidelines for activities which are effective and which meet the patient's needs. The basis for discussion is a situation wherein three nurses acted differently in response to a patient's request.

A Patient Requests an Abdominal Binder

Mrs. D. occupied the bed her nurse was making. Her eyes were focused on the abdomen of a patient in the next bed where another nurse was applying an abdominal binder. Suddenly, Mrs. D. pointed to the binder and said, "Can I please have a binder like hers?" Mrs. D.'s nurse was gathering the soiled bedclothes when a doctor appeared and asked her, "Did that report come back?" "Isn't it on the desk? I'll be right there," replied Mrs. D.'s nurse. The doctor left as the nurse answered Mrs. D., "You don't need one—you didn't have an operation like hers." Mrs. D. stared at the bedclothes as the nurse hastily left the room. Two seconds later a third nurse entered. As she handed

Mrs. D. a medication cup, Mrs. D. asked, "Nurse, can I have a binder on my belly?" As the third nurse replied, "You had a normal, spontaneous delivery—you don't need one," the first nurse returned with clean towels and interjected, "I told you, you didn't need one." Suddenly Mrs. D.'s eyes dropped as she rubbed her lips together and picked at the nail of her little finger with her thumb. Both nurses who explained that the patient didn't need a binder left the room.

The nurse who applied the binder to the other patient was now free. As she approached Mrs. D.'s bedside, she said, "I heard you ask for a binder. Can you tell me why, because we usually don't use them unless you've had an operation?" "Well, when my breasts were all swollen and the nurse wrapped them up tight, it helped them go down. I don't like this big belly I have now after the baby, and I figured if I wrapped it up tight it would go down too."

The nurse understood what the request meant and the explanation the patient needed. The nurse explained the differences in the *"swelling."* In order for the nurse to measure the effect of the explanation, she asked, "Do you still think the binder will help?" "Oh, no, I understand you—it won't help. Isn't there something that will make this belly go down?" The patient was taught postpartum exercises and did them successfully.

All three nurses had similar data. They heard the patient's request, knew their response to it and knew that the patient did not have a Caesarian section. The nurses correctly understood the routine use of abdominal binders.

The patient's request provoked the verbal activity of all three nurses. The automatic thoughts of all three had to do with the routine use of abdominal binders. Presumably the purpose of their verbal activity was also the same—to have the patient understand that she did not need a binder. One nurse decided to carry out her purpose by explaining that the patient did not have an operation; another by explaining that the patient had a normal spontaneous delivery. A third explained why it was not indicated, but added a question which explored the request, and thus found out the specific explanation the patient needed in order to understand that a binder was not indicated. Explaining the differences in the *"swelling"* enabled the nurse to achieve her purpose and thus to help the patient.

It was clear to the nurses that the patient did not actually need a binder at the time she requested it. However, the patient assumed that a binder would make *"her belly go down."* This incorrect idea had to be elicited before the nurse could discover the patient's need. The patient needed to have the thought upon which the request was based corrected. This was not automatically clear to the patient or the nurse until she discussed and thought the matter through with Mrs. D.

An examination of what happened to each nurse will focus attention on the three conditions which distinguish automatic ineffective activities from deliberative effective ones.

Initially all three nurses explained in a limited way that a binder was not indicated. However, the first two decided not to supply one without first exploring for the meaning of the patients request. The third nurse, while she also explained, did explore the request for a binder before she decided not to supply one. This illustrates the first essential difference between an automatic ineffective activity and a more deliberative effective one.

It was useful for the third nurse to explore the patient's request before refusing to comply with it. On this basis, it could be said that the first two nurses *"should"* have found out why the patient requested a binder before they decided not to supply one. But this did not take place, and probably at that moment it could not have taken place. The two reasons for this reveal two more differences between automatic ineffective activities and deliberative effective ones.

When the two nurses told the patient she did not need a binder, they thought they were correct, and, strictly speaking, they were. Their refusal to supply one was a correct decision but it did not meet the patient's need. They did not stop to find out how the patient was affected by the explanation and decision although there were nonspecific indications of affect in the patient's behavior. The first nurse might have wondered why the patient made the request a second time; the second nurse might have wondered why the patient lowered her eyes and picked at her little finger. The nurse who explained the difference in the swelling did try to find out how her initial and subsequent explanations affected the patient, and she succeeded. This illustrates the second difference between ineffective and effective nursing activities.

To say that the first two nurses could have found out how their activity affected the patient does seem reasonable. However, they were not entirely free to do so—a fact which brings us to illustrate a third and crucial difference between activities which do and those which do not help the patient. The nurse who did help the patient had as her exclusive focus the patient and her needs. There were no other stimuli to distract her. The nurses who acted automatically were responding to stimuli unrelated to the process of ascertaining and meeting Mrs. D.'s immediate need. One of the nurses automatically responded to a doctor's request and to her tasks of picking up linen and bringing in towels. The other nurse was preoccupied with the task of giving out medications. The third and essential condition for effective actions is that the nurse must be free of stimuli unrelated to the process of ascertaining and meeting the immediate need of the patient.

At this point it may be said that the activity of a nurse may be automatic or deliberative, that activities have purpose and that the purpose may or may not have to do with the process of helping the patient. If the activities are carried out without exploration for the patient's need or consideration of how they affect the patient, they constitute an automatic process. If the reverse is true, they comprise a deliberative one.

In summary, an automatic process of activity is ineffective in helping the patient for one or all of the following reasons: (1) it is decided upon for reasons other than the meaning of the patient's behavior and the unmet need giving rise to it; (2) it does not enable the patient to let the nurse know how the activity affects him; (3) it is unrelated to the patient's immediate need; (4) it may occur because the nurse is not free to explore her reaction to the patient's behavior; or (5) the nurse is unaware of how her activity affects the patient.

On the other hand, activities carried out deliberatively are effective because they help the patient for the following reasons: (1) they come about after the nurse knows the meaning of the patient's behavior and the specific activity which is required to meet his need; (2) the activity is carried out in such a way that the patient is helped to inform the nurse as to how her activity affects him; (3) the specific required activity meets the patient's need and achieves the nurse's purpose of having helped the patient *(if it does not, a new activity is decided upon);* (4) the nurse is available to respond to the patient's need for help; and (5) the nurse knows how her activity affects the patient.

How does the nurse really know whether her activity has helped the patient? Her exploratory process with the patient gives her the evidence which helps form an impression. The impression grows out of whether she observes a change for the *"better"* in the behavior which was present when she started. In the illustration just cited, the interaction began with a request for an abdominal binder which seemed unreasonable, and terminated with the patient learning how to do postpartum exercises. In order for the nurse to decide that her impression is correct, she must take into account not only verbal but also nonverbal behavior. Often both types of behavior may be observed simultaneously. When the patient requested help in strengthening her abdominal muscles, she was not staring at the bedclothes or picking her little finger or making the same request over again. Noting the consistency between the patient's verbal and nonverbal behavior made it possible for the nurse to be certain that she had helped the patient. In contrast to the consistency in Mrs. D.'s behavior is the inconsistency the nurse observed in the patient who was afraid of the spinal. Even though the activity *(telling the patient she was going to the O.R.)* was decided upon with the patient and the patient thanked the nurse, the nurse noted that her mouth and hands quivered even more than they did when the interaction started.

The nurse, therefore, knew she had not yet helped the patient and so pursued her exploration of the new observations with the patient.

Sometimes the patient's verbal confirmation that he has been helped may be misunderstood by the nurse. This can be illustrated by the patient with the stitch pain who thanked the nurse and said he felt better before she had carried out the actions which would have relieved his pain. In this situation, the nurse had to recognize clearly that the patient was relieved of the feeling that he might be crazy, not that his feeling better meant his pain was relieved. The nurse arrived at this recognition when she explored with the patient the true meaning of his last remarks.

The observation of some consistency between verbal and nonverbal behavior would seem necessary for the nurse to know whether she has helped the patient. It is also important for her to know exactly which activity was helpful. Admittedly, this is not an absolute criterion, but it is realistic for the practice of nursing. What the outcome is from the particular patient's point of view can be ascertained only from the exploration of the nurse's reaction to the patient's behavior after she thinks she has helped him. If she has not yet helped or if the patient requires additional help, then the patient can let her know.

There are then three possible ways for the patient to be affected by nursing activities—the activity may help, may not help, or the result may be unknown. Consideration of these possibilities in the light of the patient's inability to communicate clearly without help makes possible the formulation of a third nursing principle which guides the nurse when acting with or for the patient. *The nurse initiates a process of exploration to ascertain how the patient is affected by what she says or does.* Only in this way can she be clearly aware of how and whether her actions are helping the patient.

In the foregoing pages elements of nursing process were identified, analyzed and discussed. Principles crucial to the meeting of patient needs and to the nurse's effective functioning were formulated.

The fact that the nurse can perceive what is relevant or irrelevant, think correctly or incorrectly, feel appropriately or inappropriately and, further, act helpfully or harmfully, indicates that the actions and reactions of the nurse must be disciplined to become relevant, correct, appropriate and helpful to the patient. To show how this can be done, a deliberative nursing process will be described. This process makes allowances for the unique character of any nurse-patient situation and is based on the formulations of professional nursing function and principles of effective practice.

A deliberative nursing process has elements of continuous reflection as the nurse tries to understand the meaning to the patient of the behavior she observes and what he needs from her in order to be helped. Responses comprising this process are stimulated by the nurse's unfolding awareness of the particulars of the individual situation.

The nurse perceives, thinks, feels and acts according to the way she experiences her own participation in the nurse-patient situation. In each instance she has to find out more about her own action and reaction in order to understand its distinct meaning to the patient. Because of this, her responses follow a definite sequence. First, she shares with the patient aspects of her perceptions, thoughts and feelings by expressing in words or nonverbal gestures or tones her wondering, thinking, or questioning in order to learn how accurate or adequate her reaction is. The response of the patient gives rise to fresh reactions which she continues to express and explore. She must do this so that both can find out what each is thinking, and why, so that an understanding of the patient's need can be arrived at. When the patient's need is clearly discerned, the nurse can decide on an appropriate course of action. The nurse then does or says something with or for the patient, or together they decide that the help of another person is required. Whatever the action, the nurse asks the patient about it in order to find out how her action affects him.

The deliberative nursing process is clearly related to the nurse's professional function of helping the patient because she is in the position of knowing what is happening and whether or not she is being helpful. The nurse recognizes if she has met the patient's need for help by noting the presence or absence of improvement in his presenting behavior. In the absence of improvement, the nurse knows the patient's need has not yet been met, and, if she remains available, she starts the process all over again with whatever presenting behavior is then observed.

4

Problems in Nursing Situations

THE DEVELOPMENT OF NURSING PROBLEMS

Establishing a nurse-patient relationship which is dynamic is not as complicated as we may be led to believe. Discussion of previous material has pointed this out. This does not mean that the psychodynamics of the relationship are simple. They are exceedingly complex and for this reason the material was not analyzed from that point of view. However, attention has been focused on the particulars of the nurse-patient situation which were immediately relevant to one nurse's process of helping one patient. This focus has been useful, not only because knowledge of the particulars brought about the necessary understanding in the situation, but also because the understanding was achieved through whatever awareness or lack of understanding the nurse and patient had at the onset of their interaction. The guidelines for mutual understanding made it possible to bring clarity into some of the obscure complexity and in unique situations it opened the way for a fresh process of deliberation. In addition, this focus was realistic to the practical aspects of individual nurse-patient situations.

On one hand, the nurse responds not only with her own individuality, but also with a correct understanding of the purpose of the activities she performs—purposes which are not automatically understood by the patient and activities which do not automatically suit the requirements of the patient's need. On the other hand, the patient behaves in his individual way and the meaning of his behavior or the need giving rise to it is not automatically communicated to the nurse. If this is relevant to nurse-patient settings in general, then the automatic inadequate communications between the patient and the nurse are what complicate the nurse-patient situation. This phenomenon has direct bearing on the development of nursing problems. In this chapter it will be observed that the nurse is faced with problematic situations when she does not apply the principles of effective practice identified in Chapter 3.

It has been established that an activity designed for the patient's benefit may not turn out to be helpful to him. This prompts the question, "Why was it carried out in the first place?" It is common to receive the following kinds of answers to questions which ask why the nurse said or did what she did to or for the patient: "It was time to do it." "That's what I would say." "Because the patient asked for it." "The doctor ordered it." "The supervisor told me to." While such answers may reflect a misunderstanding of the nurse's function—they do not reflect the attitude of the nurse which is a fundamentally helpful one. An appropriate answer would be, "I did or said this because the patient needed it."

Regardless of the reasons the nurse offers for activities she carries out with patients, it must be assumed that her intention is to be of help. It is most unlikely that a professional nurse would ever refuse to meet a patient's need provided that she understands the need correctly. In the subsequent discussion emphasis will be placed on the fundamentally helpful attitude of the nurse. This attitude is not only commendable and consistent with the tradition and goals of nursing, but is one which can be turned to advantage by everyone interested in improving the practice of others.

Since a nurse's activity is professional only when it deliberatively achieves the purpose of helping the patient, the activity *per se* is not the decisive criterion by which it may be evaluated. Rather, what is relevant and significant is whether and how the activity serves to help the patient communicate his needs and how it is directed to their being met. While this may be accepted as a frame of reference, we must remain aware that the current organization of nursing responsibility *(in some settings)* requires or expects the nurse to carry out activities unrelated to the professional task at hand. As the number of nonprofessional duties increase, the nurse's freedom to help the patient necessarily decreases. Preoccupation with these other tasks makes the nurse less readily available to help patients with their needs. Yet, the patient's requirements for the nurse's help are essential to his welfare as well as to her effective professional functioning.

While a discussion of nonprofessional activities is unrelated to the purposes of this book, they deserve to be mentioned in order to point out that, while a nurse may carry out all kinds of activities, professional or not, she can only carry out one at a time. It seems wasteful for professionally trained nursing personnel to devote any of their time to activities other than those directly related to their function.

Professional activities are designed and carried out for the benefit of the patient. Attention will be focused on those specifically related to his care. In the previous discussion of activities it was said that decisions to act may be made with or without the patient's participation. When the nurse, in collaboration with the patient, ascertained what would meet the patient's need and acted upon it, his behavior or condition improved. It is apparent that such outcomes are unproblematic. In the same discussion it was noted that activities decided upon without adequate exploration were inconsistent with the patient's need. It could not be otherwise at the onset of an interaction. To expect the activity to suit the patient without deliberation is not realistic. How can two people know what is required from each other, except by chance, without an exchange of information? Each, just prior to their experience together, was perceiving, thinking, feeling and behaving differently. There is likely to be, at the start, an almost inevitable conflict between an automatic process of activity and the patient's immediate need. This may be described as a *"situational conflict."*

The outcome of a nursing situation depends upon the action taken by the nurse. These outcomes may or may not be helpful to the patient, or it may not be known how the patient was affected. When the patient's behavior does not show a change for the better, the nurse may assume that she is not acting effectively. The action of the nurse makes, solves, or prevents a problem.

Investigation bears out that problems arising in nursing situations are a direct result of activities decided and acted upon without taking into account the patient's immediate need. These activities are either medically prescribed or are decided upon by the nurse independently. Activities carried out without due consideration for the patient's need are also referred to as automatic in this discussion.

A few words should be said about medically prescribed activities. It is important to recognize that the nurse is using a doctor's order for the patient and is not carrying out orders for the doctor. This is logical, since, if the patient were able to carry out the diagnostic or treatment plan alone, in all probability the nurse would not become involved in the first place.

A position was taken earlier that the problems a nurse faces are not related to her desire or capacity to be helpful. Then where do her "troubles" begin? They begin with the inadequacies inherent in nursing situations, *i.e., the automatic reactions and actions of the nurse and patient and the resulting unclear communications.* When the nurse does not abide by the principles of effective practice which resolve these inadequacies, she acts automatically and allows the *"situational conflict"* to continue. In this discussion it shall be shown how this conflict comes about and the importance of resolving it at the onset of an interaction to avoid *"making"* a problem. Although problems in nurse-patient situations stem from the unresolved *"situational conflict"* they come to the attention of the nurse in one of two ways. She either finds that her activities are ineffective in bringing about the desired results or she independently decides the patient's manifest behavior is *"ineffective"* in relation to his well being. In both types of problems the helpful nature of the nurse-patient relationship becomes disrupted.

Ineffective Nursing Activities

For two reasons, ineffective activities are necessarily nursing problems. The patient allows the nurse to act in a way which is not helpful to him, and the nurse does not achieve her professional purpose.

Four illustrations will be used as a basis for this discussion. In each, the following points may be noted: (1) the activity designed or intended for the patient's benefit, but carried out automatically, is ineffective; (2) the automatic activity is ineffective because the patient's immediate need was not ascertained and met; and (3) if the automatic activity is not redirected through a process of reflection, then a whole series of ineffective actions result which further delay improvement in the patient's condition.

Nurses Administer Codeine for a Headache

"Nurse, I have a very bad headache," said the patient who squinted as she tried to sit up. She supported her weight with one hand and with the other held her head as if to protect it from moving in relation to her body. The nurse automatically assumed the patient needed what the doctor ordered *(codeine gr. i; aspirin gr. x)* to relieve her headache.

"Here are your pills; they'll take about 20 minutes to work," said the nurse before she left the room. It was 10 A.M. Two hours later the patient complained again, "My headache is very bad." The nurse said, "It isn't time for your medicine. You still have two hours to go." The nurse, in leaving the room, said to another, "She can hardly see straight." The other nurse reviewed the notes and saw that the patient had received codeine gr. i and aspirin gr. x every four hours for *"severe headache"* for the two previous days.

The patient's eyes were closed as she held on to her temples. "I just found out that this is the third day you have had a headache. The pills we've been giving you don't seem to help it—do they?" The patient opened, then closed her eyes as if to nod, put both hands up to the back of her neck and started to rub it. The nurse explored this new nonverbal response by asking "Why are you doing that?" The patient replied, "It soothes it." "Since it sounds better than the pills, can I help you do it?" The patient said, "Would you please, nurse?"

As the nurse massaged the back of the patient's neck, the patient exclaimed, "Oh . . . how good that feels!" In order to know the effect of the pressure and the rubbing, the nurse asked about it after several strokes. Some of the patient's replies were: "Keep it up." "The harder you rub the better it feels." "I'll tell you when it hurts . . . just keep it up." After about five minutes of massage, the patient spontaneously put her hand up and said, "Stop a minute . . ." She shook her head, then said, "I think it's gone . . . I can't believe it!" Abruptly she sat up, shook her head more vigorously from side to side as if something incredible had happened, then said, "I can't believe it . . . it's been killing me for three days. What do you think of that? All I needed was a massage."

The next morning as the nurse passed the patient's room, the patient called out, "How can I ever thank you? I had a good night's sleep last night. About midnight I felt the headache coming back, but I called the night nurse and she knew what you did and how much it helped; she rubbed my neck for two minutes and that was it. The headache didn't come back again."

Nurses Administer Medication for a Patient's
Blood Pressure

For a period of one week nurses administered an intramuscular medication every hour for the reduction of a patient's blood pressure. On this particular morning, before each injection the blood pressure remained stable at 182/118.

In the afternoon of the same day, the head nurse asked another nurse, "Would you give her the intramuscular? I just checked her blood pressure—it's 182/118. There is almost no point in taking it—it's been the same all week." The nurse then realized that the medication was not helping the patient. She said to the patient,

"The head nurse tells me your blood pressure hasn't changed much, and it's hard for me to understand why, because these injections should help." "I think I know why, nurse, but I don't want to say anything—everyone here is very good to me." "What's that have to do with your blood pressure?" "I don't want to say it, but I think it's the injections that make it go up." The nurse wondered about this. "I lie here every hour day and night worrying because they hurt and burn. I'm a nervous wreck when it's time for the needle. I really think it's my nerves, and, when it's time for them to take my blood pressure, it's always up." To make sure that she understood the patient correctly, the nurse asked, "You mean you are nervous waiting for the injections and that keeps your pressure up?" The patient nodded and said, "Yes, nurse." "Well, what you say makes sense to me. I wonder if you can pretend that I won't give you the needle the next hour, because, if the pressure does come down, you won't have to have it." "Yes, yes . . . thanks . . . nurse, I'm sure it will be down."

When the hour was up the patient's blood pressure was 140/80, a reading which did not require the intramuscular. The hourly blood pressure checks for the rest of the day showed that the blood pressure remained stable between 136/88 and 140/80.

Nurses Carry Out Prescribed Activities to Facilitate a Patient's Bowel Movement

The patient complained of *"cramps"* for three days because of her inability to have a bowel movement. Because of this, she was not discharged on the regular postpartum day.

During the three days, nurses assumed that the patient required all that the doctor ordered, *i.e., three enemas, two suppositories, and milk of magnesia at bedtime.* Fluids were forced. Pain medication gave the patient some relief.

On the fourth day, the night nurse reported, "She was awake all night. She's in agony . . . her pain medication has not helped." The day nurse reflected on the ineffective nursing activities and decided that the patient required something other than what the nurses had been doing.

The nurse entered the patient's room and said, "Nothing we have done has helped you feel better or have a bowel movement, do you agree?" The patient looked up, hesitated, looked away, but did not speak. "Were you going to say something?" "Aren't they supposed to give you an enema before you have your baby?" replied the patient. "They usually do. Didn't you have one?" The patient burst into tears and through her sobbing said, "How horrible it was . . . the delivery was nothing . . . but trying to hold the bowel movement in and push the baby out at the same time was living hell." The nurse wondered aloud about the physiological *"impossibility"* of what happened to the patient. "I would rather have died than have a bowel movement in that position with everybody looking," the patient added. The patient continued to cry, and as she did the nurse expressed her amazement again by saying, "I still can't understand how you were able to manage it." The patient dried her eyes and sighed deeply, then said, "I didn't realize it before, but I think that's why I've been so tight inside . . . can I have a bedpan now?" The patient had her bowel movement.

Nurses Explain to the Patient Why She Won't
Bleed to Death

A patient had a Caesarian section the previous night. The night nurse reported, "She spent the whole night checking her perineal pad—she's afraid she is going to bleed to death. I explained why she won't, but she continues to check the pad. I don't know what's wrong with her."

The day nurse had cared for the patient on and off during three previous admissions when the patient was threatening placenta previa. The same day nurse entered the patient's room. The patient turned her head toward the doorway and with one finger in her mouth, stared at the nurse. Suddenly, she released her finger and strained her neck to look at her perineal pad. While the nurse walked to the bedside, the patient checked the pad two more times.

"I see you looking at your pad—how come?" "I want to be sure I don't bleed to death." Automatically the nurse assumed the patient required an explanation and told her why the doctors were no longer concerned about bleeding. The explanation was ineffective because the patient continued checking. The nurse tried to explain the point further by describing the physiology of the uterus.

While the nurse gathered bath equipment, she realized that the patient required something other than what she had already said because the patient kept checking the pad. "The explanations I gave you don't seem to help, do they?" "Of course not, if nobody checks, then I've got to." "As far as I know we don't have to, but why do you say we should?" The patient burst forth with, "Then what's that sheet of paper hanging on the door? They write on it often enough, but they don't check my pad, and that's all they did when I was here before."

The sheet the patient referred to had vital signs recorded on it. The sheet used during previous admissions, which was also posted on the door, was used to record the pad count.

The nurse told the patient that she now understood why the patient was checking, and proceeded to explain the differences in the posted sheets of paper. The patient sighed and said, "Everybody told me I wasn't going to bleed to death, but I didn't believe them. I thought they were lying. They wrote on the sheet, but they didn't check my pad like they used to." The patient stopped checking.

In approximately a 10-minute period during one of the patient's previous admissions, two doctors stopped at the door of her room to look at the posted sheet which had the pad count on it. One glanced over to the patient and they exchanged greetings. About two minutes later the head nurse came, looked at the same sheet of paper on the door, removed it, examined the patient's pad and then placed a new sheet on the door. Four minutes later the nurse assigned to the patient approached the bedside and said, "Let me see, have you used any pads since the last one I gave you?" The patient shook her head, indicating no. The nurse inspected the pad and made a notation.

These illustrations point up rather clearly the conflict between the specific activity the patient requires from the nurse in order to be helped and the automatic activities which are assumed to be needed. For example, one patient required a neck rub, not codeine; another needed information about a sheet posted on her door, not an explanation as to why the doctors were no longer concerned about her bleeding; another needed to tell the nurse why she was *"tight"* inside, but she did not need cathartics; still another needed to know that she would not be given an intramuscular. These examples are not intended to question the reasonableness of the nurses' assumptions that their activities would be helpful. Each activity was in accord with medical orders and with principles which explain why they were carried out—codeine may relieve a headache; a specific medication may reduce an elevated blood pressure; cathartics may facilitate a bowel movement; an explanation of why placenta previa will not cause bleeding after delivery may relieve a patient's fear.

It is not suggested that nurses have jurisdiction over medical orders. These are decisions geared to the medical needs of patients and are, therefore, the responsibility of the physician. He alone has the prerogative to prescribe. However, in current nursing practice, the nurse carries out prescribed activities and is doing so for the benefit of the patient. While her activity is medically prescribed in these instances, her use of the order would necessarily take into consideration the responsibility inherent in any act a nurse performs with or for the patient, *i.e., it would consider how the activity affects the patient.* Regardless of whether the nurse finds the activity helpful or not, she does not change what is prescribed. Instead, she informs the doctor about the results of the prescribed activity and, if he does not yet know them, he continues, changes, or cancels his orders as he deems necessary.

The four illustrations just cited point up again that the patient's behavior does not improve until principles of effective nursing practice are applied.

Any automatic activity is ineffective unless the nurse finds out that the patient was in fact helped by it. If the nurse finds out that the activity has not helped, she can redirect her attention to further exploration for the purpose of finding out what specific activity will meet the patient's need. If the nurse does not reflect on how her actions affect the patient, then the patient's unmet need stands in the way of any improvement in his condition. It can be concluded then that ineffective activities may be prevented if the nurse ascertains and meets the patient's need before making any decisions as to which activity is indicated.

Ineffective Patient Behavior

Ineffective patient behavior is used to mean any behavior which prevents the nurse from carrying out her concerns for the patient's care or from maintaining a satisfactory relationship to the patient. These behaviors are often termed *"uncooperative," "unreasonable," "demanding,"* or *"commanding."*

When the patient refuses to cooperate, he prevents the nurse from carrying out activities which are designed for his benefit, and thus he behaves in a way which is seemingly inconsistent with his well being. When he makes unreasonable requests, or demands, or spends most of his time commanding the nurse, he behaves in a way which can prevent the nurse from liking him. In a sense, when the patient behaves in a way which makes the nurse think he is unreasonable, then the behavior is in direct opposition to the nurse's prerogatives in carrying out her professional function of helping him. When he *"commands"* or is *"unreasonable,"* he is not recognizing the professional nurse's *"know how."* Commands and demands are generally issued to a person only when that person is, or is thought to be, unwilling to comply.

It might be useful here to repeat one statement concerning the patient's presenting behavior. Regardless of its form, *e.g., requests, refusals, demands,* the nurse must view it as a possible signal of distress or a manifestation of an unmet need.

The discussion of the patient's ineffective behavior will highlight the same points made in connection with ineffective nursing activities: (1) if the initial *"situational conflict"* is not resolved, the nurse has a problem to deal with; (2) the problem comes about because the activity designed and intended for the patient's benefit but carried out automatically is ineffective; (3) the activity is ineffective because the patient's need was not ascertained and met; and (4) if the activity is not redirected through a process of reflection, a series of ineffective activities may result and further delay improvement in the patient's condition. In each of the subsequent illustrations, when principles of effective practice are applied the nurse is able to ascertain and meet the patient's immediate need, thereby changing the patient's ineffective behavior and resolving the nursing problem.

A Patient Refuses an Intravenous

The nurse entered with an intravenous tray. Abruptly, the patient sat up and yelled, "Get out of here! Nobody, but nobody is going to put that needle in me today. You people will drive me nuts." The nurse said, "I'm sorry, but it's ordered daily." The patient replied, "I don't give a damn—get it out of here. The nurse placed the tray on the bedside table, left the room, approached the head nurse and said, "The patient refuses her infusion and she really sounds like she means it." The head nurse responded, "I'll go in and talk with her."

The head nurse said to the patient, "You have to have the intravenous—it's ordered daily . . . there isn't enough fluid in your body . . ." The patient interrupted, "I'm not listening. If you don't get that tray out of here, I'll throw it through the window." The head nurse bit her lip and said, "O.K., I'll see what the doctor says."

Another nurse immediately approached the patient and said, "You really look upset. Can you tell me why?" The patient started to cry, then said, "Wouldn't you be upset if the doctor promised you that if you drank all night you wouldn't get the intravenous? I stayed awake drinking all night. I'm floating now. What more do they want from me?"

The fluid intake notes confirmed the patient's achievement. The doctor was notified and the order for intravenous was discontinued.

A Patient Requests, Then Demands, To Go Home

During the first hospital day, a patient blurted out, "Nurse, I asked everybody in a nice way if I could go home and they tell me no, because I'm on observation. If you tell me I can't, too, then I'm just going to walk out of here even if I have to go without my clothes." "Why do you want to go home?" "I have to or my house will blow up. I left the water heater on high and no one is there to turn it off. I'm the only one that has a key. If it stays up high after today, the house will blow to hell." "Is this the only reason you want to go home?" "Yes, what do you think I came to the hospital for? I want to stay—it's just the hot water heater."

The nurse said, "Isn't there someone else who could do it?" "Yes, nurse, I have a girl friend. I'm sure she'll come and get the key, but she's got to know about it. I asked if I could use the telephone this morning to call her, but they told me I wasn't allowed out of bed. Will you call her for me? I know she'll come to the hospital for the key."

The friend agreed to come within the hour. The patient replied when the nurse informed him, "What a relief! Now I can relax."

A Patient Refuses a Pill

As the nurse was about to hand a patient a Dicumarol tablet, she said, "I have a pill for you." The patient said, "Let's see it." The nurse placed the pill within the patient's view. "You're crazy, I'm not going to take that." The nurse flushed and left the room. Another nurse asked the patient, "Can you tell me why you won't take your pill?" "Because I took one just a minute ago." "Who gave it to you?" "Myself—I brought my own Dicumarol with me. It was time to take it and I did."

These situations point out on the one hand that, as long as the nurse allows the patient to behave *"ineffectively,"* the problem remains. Not only did the ineffective behavior continue, but in all likelihood it would have become more intense until the situation was clarified. It was imperative that one patient not receive an intravenous, that the other get his water heater turned off and that the third patient not take a second Dicumarol pill. The patients' behavior, while seemingly ineffective to the nurses, really represented the struggle against what they did not need or their struggle to get their needs met. They were frustrated in their attempts to meet their own needs in their own ways, as happened to the patient who drank until she *"floated"* so that she wouldn't get an intravenous, and to the patient who asked if he could make a telephone call to prevent his house from blowing up. The third patient took his Dicumarol on time and refused a second one for a good and adequate reason.

At this point the illustrations cited may seem too simple and illustrate only the use of common sense. However, the situations were not simple to start with. The patients talked to the nurses angrily and insistently, in methods of address that would not ordinarily provoke another to respond warmly and helpfully. Simplification of the situations grew out of the nurse's awareness that the presenting behavior was a manifestation of the patient's unmet need. She realized at the onset that the patient's ineffective behavior was not directed to her as a person, but to an automatic activity which did not suit his need—the setting up of an intravenous; the offering of a pill; the refusal of a patient's urgent request to use the phone.

Thus, the ineffective behavior of the patient may initially seem to be in direct opposition to the nurse's interest in him. By stopping to find out what is wrong, the nurse is able to understand that the patient does not really oppose her but that his need is not being met.

In case these situations seem too simple to account for the *"big"* nursing problems, one may be reported that on the surface seemed *"greater."* Again the root of the problem was the same, that is, the initial conflict between the patient's immediate need and the automatic activity was not resolved by the nurse.

In this problem the patient and the nurse could not get together to achieve their common purpose. The patient refused emphatically to do postural drainage. The nurse knew how important it was for the patient to do so, but the patient's insistent refusal frustrated nurses for four days and drastically interfered with his improvement.

A Patient Refuses to Do Postural Drainage

At morning report the night nurse said, "He still won't do his postural drainage and he's getting more and more negative about it." The head nurse said to the staff nurse who was assigned to care for the patient, "You must get him to do it today—at least once. It's been four whole days and his lung congestion is getting worse by the minute."

Twenty minutes later a nurse saw the patient from the hall. He was sitting in bed, his face was blue, and he seemed to be exerting a great deal of effort in breathing. The nurse assigned to the patient entered and said, "It's time for you to do your postural drainage." Abruptly the patient interrupted, "I told you people a hundred times . . . that I'm not going to do it. Air has to go in here *(pointing to his chest)* or you don't live." As the nurse shook her head, she said, "You won't do it?" "I said I wouldn't. Don't you understand English?" The nurse sighed, turned abruptly and left the room. The nurse who was watching from the hall entered and expressed one aspect of what she thought, "It looks as though you're having trouble breathing, are you?" "That's right, nurse. That's what I'm in the hospital for." "Has being in the hospital made it better or worse?" The patient shook his head and said, "It's worse, nurse. The doctors and nurses keep telling me it's because I won't do the postural drainage, but I don't care what anybody says, I'm not going to do it."

"Can you tell me why you won't do it?" "Because I can't; it's too uncomfortable—but that's not the half of it. When I lean over the chair with my head upside down, the chair hits me here in the pit of my stomach. All the weight of my body is on it, and it's impossible for me to breathe, let alone cough. I wouldn't mind half as much if it helped me to cough, but it doesn't at all that way. I cough better when I'm sitting up."

The nurse then said, "It certainly makes sense not to do it that way if it doesn't help you to cough. I know of a different position that keeps your head at an angle but not upside down and doesn't put all the weight on your stomach. However, even this position is usually uncomfortable." "Even if it is, nurse, I'd like to try it. It's very hard to breathe this way . . . I want to cough some up but I can't over that chair."

For each direction the nurse gave the patient she asked how it felt. Each time the patient responded differently. For instance, "This is all right. This is no strain. So far, so good, etc. . . ." The nurse noted that these responses were inconsistent with his color, which seemed purple, and with his even more difficult breathing. "Even though you say it's all right, you seem worse now. Are you?" "No, I said it's good!" "Can I give you some oxygen then?" "Yes, that ought to take care of what you think." The nurse turned on the oxygen. The patient took a deep breath and started to cough more and more vigorously. Through his cough, he said, "It's working . . . I'm coughing." The nurse commented, "You look even bluer now. Do you feel worse?" The patient's coughing prevented his responding for about a half a minute. He then said, "This is easy . . . Even though it's torture, I can take this for a half hour easy." The patient told the nurse when he did and did not need her help for oxygen and tissues. Twenty minutes passed; the nurse remarked, "It seems to me you have worked hard enough for this first time .. . . no?" "Yeah, I think so too; let me rest now." When he had assumed a resting position, the nurse arranged the pillows and gave the patient more oxygen until he said, "I don't need the oxygen now, I'm better." The nurse thought so too.

About an hour later the patient called out to the nurse who at that moment was passing in the hall, "Say, nurse, I feel better in every way. I'm breathing easier and I feel good now. I coughed up a lot, didn't I?"

The nurse said reflectively, "You know, it's ordered three times a day, and I'm wondering if it will be as hard for you to do it twice more since it looked so tough the first time." Sure I can . . . It wasn't hard. It was the position over the chair that I couldn't get into no matter what."

This patient at the beginning of the interaction behaved as though he did not want to do what would benefit him. This example leads to the conclusion that the problems brought about by refusals to cooperate can be resolved if the nurse ascertains and meets the patient's need.

An understanding of ineffective activities and the time they may entail can have some relevance to the current nursing shortage. Aside from the time used in the direct contact with the patient, additional time is spent in preparation for the activity. Any one of the previous illustrations may serve to illustrate this point. For example, one patient received a total of 13 doses of codeine for severe headache, none of which helped. Allowing a total of five minutes per nurse per dose, the invested time is 65 minutes. It is apparent that five minutes per dose is a minimum amount of time, since each administration necessarily entailed checking the medical order, counting the remaining tablets, charting the dose in the narcotic book and in the patient's chart, and answering the patient's complaint. Time was consumed in walking to and from the patient's room. Some time was also used as the nurses verbally reported the headache to each other, as well as in ordering and signing for the supply of narcotics. On the other hand, the activity of both nurses who rubbed the patient's neck took significantly less time in relation to the end result. The first nurse spent about five minutes rubbing the patient's neck, and the second nurse presumably took two. Even allowing some time for the nurses to walk to and from the patient's room and for the verbal interaction with the patient, the total time for both nurses probably did not exceed 15 minutes.

Ineffective activities may also have other important implications, *e.g., the cost of nursing care, the progress of the patient's condition, the cost of materials, drugs, and the like*—all of which may be challenging areas for study by those interested in these problems.

The discussion of nursing problems has helped to demonstrate the importance of ascertaining and meeting the patient's immediate need at the onset of interaction before an activity is decided upon. It can be noted that when such deliberation did not take place, the problems which resulted were in effect direct results of the patient's unmet needs. These problems came to the attention of the nurse when her activities did not achieve the desired results or when the patient's behavior seemed *"ineffective"* in the interests of his own well being.

The next topic for consideration is methods of resolving or preventing problems in order that the nurse may work effectively as she goes about establishing, maintaining, or reestablishing the helpful nature of her direct relationship to the patient.

METHODS OF PREVENTION AND RESOLUTION

The methods of prevention and resolution discussed here are no different from the others previously discussed because the same deliberative process is involved.

Whether or not a problem is prevented or resolved is really a question of timing. If the nurse acts without resolving the initial *"situational conflict," (that is, carries out an automatic activity rather than one directed toward the patient's need),* a problem ensues. If the nurse first resolves the *situational conflict,* then she forestalls the development of a problem. Although an automatic activity may accidentally suit the requirements of the patient, decisions to act without due consideration of the patient's need are ineffective and lead to new problems. However, it is most important to plan and decide on certain activities long before the interaction takes place, or for that matter long before the patient comes to the hospital. This is particularly true in relation to routines of patient care *(serving food, evening care, morning care, etc.),* routines which protect the interests and safety of the patient *(locking doors, adjusting side rails, protecting the patient's property, restricting visitors, observing isolation procedures, aseptic technique, etc.)* and routines which protect the organization *(obtaining the patient's permission for operative procedures, and signatures for releases).*

While these routines are necessary, they are automatic activities and as such the nurse must maintain an awareness of the possible repercussions. In maintaining such awareness, she has two ways of dealing with automatic activities. First she may act or attempt to act, and then find out whether the patient was helped or at least not distressed by it. If the patient was not helped, she has a problem and must then go on to ascertain the specific activity which is required. A second way is for her to hold her decision to act in abeyance and first ascertain the patient's immediate need, thereby preventing a problem. Although it was stated earlier that the latter method is better for the patient and more appropriate to the nurse's effective functioning, both possibilities are given because in some situations the nurse may have no alternative but to act automatically.

In the following situation the nurse carried out an automatic activity which was *"right"* for her to carry out but which distressed the patient. However, the patient's distress was relieved when the nurse redirected her activity in collaboration with the patient.

A Nurse Directs the Patient to Get a Voucher in
Order to Administer Penicillin

A nurse said to a patient who sat in the clinic waiting room, "You look exhausted. Are you?" The patient shook her head rapidly and said, "No, I just came for penicillin. I'm not supposed to see the doctor or anything. I've been waiting for two hours."

The nurse then went on to say, "I think you can have the penicillin without having to wait, but I don't know for sure. What if we ask the head nurse?" "Yes, please."

In the patient's presence the nurse asked the head nurse, "Does this patient have to wait? She's only here for penicillin." "Oh, no," said the head nurse, "bring her here—she can have it now." A broad smile crossed the patient's face as she followed the head nurse, who at that moment asked, "Where is your voucher?" *(The voucher was an authorization that the state welfare department would defray the cost of the penicillin.)* The patient stopped short; the smile left her face. She stared at the head nurse, then suddenly dropped her eyes as she said, "I don't have one, nurse." The patient continued to stare at the floor as the head nurse said, "The pharmacy won't give you penicillin unless you have a voucher. You'll have to go down-town to your social worker to get one." The patient nodded as she held her mouth with her hand, turned and started to walk away. The nurse held the patient by the arm to prevent her leaving and asked, "Will you be able to get the voucher?" The patient nodded. The nurse still thought the patient looked ex-hausted and said, "You don't look as if you can go, can you?" "Well, I left my children home with a neighbor. I told her I'd be back shortly because I only had to come for the injection, and I'm late now. I'm worried because my little one should be fed, and I don't know if my neighbor knows. Besides, the other two are sick. They have chicken-pox. My neighbor is very helpful, and I don't want to take advantage of her."

The head nurse immediately said, "If that's the case, I can give it to you from stock today. Will you bring me two vouchers next time you come? I must have them." "Yes, nurse, I'll bring two day after tomorrow when I come for my next injection." While the head nurse administered the penicillin, the patient said, "You nurses are so very nice . . . thanks . . . I could never have made it downtown and back today." The head nurse responded, "I'm just glad we found out that it would be so hard for you to get the voucher today."

The appropriateness of directing the patient to get a voucher cannot be questioned. But it would have been unreasonably difficult for the patient to get the voucher. If the head nurse had not found out how the automatic direction affected the patient, there probably would have been no immediate problem for the nurse because the patient was about to leave the clinic. Yet, a problem did exist for the patient, and a problem might have developed for the nurse if the patient did not return for her penicillin.

Thus an activity may be *"correct"* when automatically carried out but ineffective in helping the patient or in obtaining the desired result. Once the activity takes place, however, the nurse may explore for its effect as a way of ascertaining the patient's need. It is possible for the nurse to find out that her automatic activity does not distress the patient, or she may learn it was incorrectly formulated and has to be redirected. In this way the nurse may resolve the problem to which an automatic activity may give rise.

To prevent problems and so that patients may better use her helpful services, the nurse may hold in abeyance any *"right"* decision to act at the onset of the interaction. One illustration of this concerns a child who had not yet learned to speak. The interaction involves a process which is deliberative except for one aspect, *i.e., the nonverbal behavior of the child.* Naturally, a child who has not yet learned to talk is unable verbally to validate or correct any aspects of the nurse's reaction. In such a case, the nurse relies exclusively on nonverbal behavior as the means of validation. The nurse acts on her perceptions, thoughts and feelings as they occur, and then looks for the results of her action.

A Nurse Decides to Feed Susan

Susan was sitting in the corner of her crib as the nurse entered with pablum and a cup of milk to feed her. As Susan looked up, the nurse thought she looked sad. The nurse picked up the child, but Susan dropped her eyes. With Susan in her lap, the nurse offered a spoonful of pablum, but Susan abruptly turned her head away. Since this was the first indication the nurse had that Susan did not want to eat, she decided to hold in abeyance what she had set out to do so that she could explore for Susan's immediate need. However, Susan's eyes remained downcast, and she did not move. The nurse thought Susan preferred the crib because she had seemed less withdrawn there. In testing out the thought, she put the child back. Immediately Susan screamed and clenched her fists. Realizing that she had been mistaken, the nurse picked Susan up again. The child stopped screaming.

In the nurse's lap again, Susan's eyes were no longer downcast, but were focused on the drawers of the bedside table. The nurse thought Susan was interested in the drawers. To see if she was right, she pulled one out. Immediately the child reached out, looked at the nurse, quickly shut the drawer and laughed. The nurse opened both drawers. Susan closed them and laughed.

The nurse opened them again. This time Susan picked up items in the drawer and let them fall. This continued for three minutes. Each time Susan moved she looked at the nurse and laughed. The nurse said as she too laughed, "If you're having such a good time now, maybe you can eat." Without interrupting the play, the nurse fed the pablum to Susan.

Whenever the nurse held the cup of milk for Susan to drink, she stopped playing to hold the cup, would drink, and then resumed playing. Susan repeated this for three more times before another nurse entered with an intramuscular injection and said, "I can't believe it. I sat with her for 30 minutes yesterday and she ate nothing."

The first nurse explored her reaction to the second nurse, "Gee, I wonder if the injection will stop her from eating. Can it wait until she finishes?" "Sure, I'll make the crib in the meantime. I'm delighted to see her eat."

The child continued playing, eating and drinking until a few drops of milk were left, at which time she shook her head from side to side, indicating to the nurse that she had had enough.

The nurse turned the child over on her lap. As she pulled the diaper down for the second nurse, she thought the injection would hurt. She reflected this thought by rubbing the child's buttock and saying, "Oh, how it's going to hurt! Oh, how it's going to hurt." The child laughed and seemed to be enjoying it thoroughly; her gurgling continued. At the moment the needle was inserted, Susan gasped, looked toward the nurse as if stunned, but did not cry. As soon as the needle came out, the nurse rubbed Susan's buttock saying, "Doesn't it hurt? Doesn't it hurt?" Susan continued her gurgling laughter. When the nurse retied the diaper, Susan continued playing. Both nurses exclaimed surprise because the child did not cry but showed an appropriate stunned look at the moment the needle was inserted. The second nurse said, "How fantastic! Yesterday she screamed and cried until she fell asleep."

Before their interactive experience started, the nurse appropriately decided to feed Susan but did not know what Susan needed at that moment. Even though the nurse automatically picked Susan up and tried to feed her, she was able to recognize that Susan did not immediately indicate a desire to eat. By holding off her decision to feed Susan and testing out the thoughts which occurred to her, she was able to discover clearly that the child needed to return to her arms. When this was done, the child was less withdrawn and indicated a desire to play, to which the nurse responded. This brought the child out so that she no longer looked sad. When the behavior of the child improved, she was able to *"cooperate"* in relation to what the nurses felt they had to do for her—to feed her and to give her an injection.

Presumably, on the previous day the second nurse had not ascertained the needs which blocked her activities from helping the child. The child ate nothing although the nurse sat for half an hour with her, and she screamed until she fell asleep after the intramuscular.

Thus, if the nurse automatically decides on the *"right"* activity but holds in abeyance what she wants to achieve until she ascertains and meets the patient's need, she helps the patient and achieves her primary objective. If the nurse is not able to carry out what she thinks is indicated, she helps the patient tell her why her judgment is inappropriate or incorrect. She then makes a new decision or continues to explore what is going on so that the patient will understand and accept what the nurse believes is indicated. In either case the purpose is to help the patient.

Another way to think of this is that either the patient is willing to go along with the nurse, or the nurse is willing to go along with the patient. They have to move together to achieve a common goal. In the situation with the Dicumarol capsule, the nurse had to go along with the patient; he did not need the medication she tried to give him. In the situation with the abdominal binder the patient had to yield to the nurse; the patient did not need a binder.

In conclusion, there is a necessary conflict between any automatic activity and the patient's immediate requirements for help. This conflict can be resolved by dealing with the subsequent problem after the activity takes place. The conflict can also be dealt with immediately if the nurse holds her decision to act in abeyance and first ascertains the patient's need, thereby preventing the problem from occurring.

Problems in the nurse-patient relationship can therefore be resolved or prevented. Whichever method the nurse uses, she can establish, maintain or re-establish her helpfulness if she initiates a process of ascertaining the patient's immediate need.

This book has not dealt with long-range nursing goals because the process of helping the patient takes place in immediate situations and the outcomes for the person being helped depend on those very experiences. However, repeated experiences of having been helped undoubtedly culminate over periods of time in greater degrees of improvement.

Cumulative effects of nursing on the improvement of the patient's condition are an exciting and fertile area for further study and investigation. It is possible to recognize cumulative effects of a deliberative nursing process through the practical experience of several nurses over a period of time with the same patient. It might be of interest to illustrate this point.

A Patient is "Scared to Death"

Following the birth of her second child, a patient was "scared to death to touch the new baby." She had had a postpartum psychosis after the birth of her first child, and this time too plans were made for her to be transferred to a state hospital on her third day postpartum. However, it turned out that the patient was not transferred. For four days nurses had explored each of the patient's presenting verbal and nonverbal behaviors in order to ascertain her immediate needs. As each need was met, the verbal manifestations of the patient's improvement progressed from "scared to death to touch the baby" to the following remarks: "Can I look at the baby while you *(the nurse)* hold her?" "Can I touch the baby's hand?" "Can I feed the baby while you *(the nurse)* hold her?" "Can I help hold the baby?" Finally, she was able to feed the baby herself provided that "you *(the nurse)* stay with me in case I get scared."

Approximately six weeks after the discharge of the patient, one of the nurses who had worked with the patient met her in the psychiatric clinic. The patient called out, "Nurse, I don't know what your name is, but I remember you. I never had a chance to thank you and the other nurses for saving my mind and giving me courage. If you had not helped me I wouldn't be coming to the clinic now. I'd be in the state mental hospital like before."

Of course, all patients cannot be helped by the nurse to this degree. Rather, the improvement is always relative to what the nurse and patient start with, to the length of their contact and to what they are able to accomplish. In each contact the nurse repeats a process of learning how to help the individual patient. Her own individuality and that of the patient require that she go through this each time she is called upon to render service to those who need her.